THE RUNNER'S WORLD® COMPLETE GUIDE TO MINIMALISM AND BAREFOOT RUNNING

THE RUNNER'S WORLD® COMPLETE GUIDE TO MINIMALISM AND BAREFOOT RUNNING

How to Make the Healthy Transition to Lightweight Shoes and Injury-Free Running

SCOTT DOUGLAS

RODALE.

© 2013 by Scott Douglas

Rodale books may be purchased for business or promotional use or for special sales.
For information, please write to:
Special Markets Department, Rodale Inc., 733 Third Avenue, New York, NY 10017.

Runner's World is a registered trademark of Rodale Inc.

Printed in the United States of America

Rodale Inc. makes every effort to use acid-free ∞, recycled paper ♲.

Book design by Christopher Rhoads

Photographs by Stacey Cramp

Library of Congress Cataloging-in-Publication Data is on file with the publisher.

ISBN–13: 978–1–60961–222–1

Distributed to the trade by Macmillan

2 4 6 8 10 9 7 5 3 1   paperback

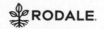

We inspire and enable people to improve their lives and the world around them.
rodalebooks.com

TO ALL
AMBITIOUS RUNNERS
WITH
OPEN MINDS

CONTENTS

THE RUNNER'S WORLD COMPLETE GUIDE TO MINIMALISM AND BAREFOOT RUNNING

CHAPTER 1

AN INTRODUCTION TO MINIMALISM

The ideas behind running in less shoe, and how this book will help you safely implement them

MARK TOMKINSON'S STORY is one you hear a lot these days.

A resident of Huntington Beach, California, Tomkinson started running in 2006. He ran half-marathons and marathons but battled injuries on and off. While training for a marathon in 2011, he had shin pain and tendinitis in his knee. Intrigued by stories of runners who'd become injury-free after switching from conventional running shoes to lower, lighter, flatter models, he ditched his old running shoes. He switched to doing all his running in a few popular minimalist shoes and barefoot. In 2012, he returned to the marathon he'd run in conventional shoes the year before and improved his time from 3:57 to 3:29. "I've gotten much faster, more efficient and 95 percent of the knee and shin problems have gone away," Tomkinson says. "I am a huge advocate of minimalist running and preach it to anyone who will listen."

Mimi Englander's story is also one you hear a lot these days.

In 2010, the Littleton, Massachusetts, resident started running in Vibram FiveFingers. At first, things went well. She was able to run 7 miles at a time, 3 miles farther than she ever had in conventional running shoes. Longtime knee, back, and bunion issues improved. She stepped up her training even more and ran her first half-marathon in FiveFingers. Then the foot pain started. She kept running. About a year into her switch to FiveFingers, she stopped running because of pain in both Achilles tendons. She got an x-ray on her painful foot and learned that she had a metatarsal stress fracture. A year later, Englander was still getting back to running. "It's slow going, as it should be," she says. "My experience hasn't dissuaded me; I know what I did wrong and am listening to my feet much more carefully, working to refine my form at the same time."

Tomkinson and Englander are two of the millions of runners who've become intrigued by minimalist and barefoot running. In the past few years, no aspect of running has been discussed more than what type and how much shoe is best. Barefoot running has gone mainstream. Minimalism, or running in something other than conventional training shoes, has spread from a small segment of competitive runners to account for 11 percent of the US running shoe market in the first quarter of 2012.

WHAT'S IT ALL ABOUT?

In the early 2000s, running message boards began to fill with complaints about the state of running shoes. Longtime runners were frustrated by most of what was commercially available. The shoes, they said, were too heavy, too high off the ground, too heeled, too full of gadgetry purported to correct flaws in people's running form. The shoes, they said, hurt rather than helped performance

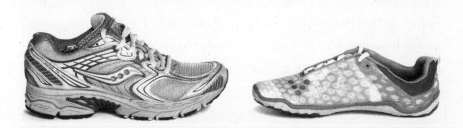

The differences between a conventional running shoe (Saucony Ride) and a minimalist shoe (Vivobarefoot Evo) are obvious when you put the shoes next to each other.

and increased rather than decreased injury rates. Runners shared experiences of switching to other types of shoes for all their mileage. Some opted for retro running shoes from the 1970s marketed as urban fashion wear. Some started doing even their slowest training runs in racing shoes. Others took a longtime practice of occasional barefoot running and did more and more of their running unshod.

The critique of modern running shoes went like this: By placing a large amount of soft foam and an elevated heel between the runner's foot and the ground, modern running shoes change people's running form for the worse. Modern shoes encourage a hard heel landing rather than a softer midfoot landing; the latter is how people run when barefoot, the critique continued. Hard heel landings are like braking with every step, which slows you down and sends the impact forces of landing up your body, leading to injury.

In addition, the critique continued, the large amounts of cushioning rob the body of its natural means of stability, because the feet can no longer get good sensory feedback as they roll through the gait cycle. Being so big, the shoes add weight that makes a quick, light cadence more difficult. The critique ended with the point that all the add-ons, like motion-control devices and midsoles of different densities, add more weight and rob the foot that much more of its ability to run naturally.

This isn't as radical a critique as it might seem at first. The type of running shoe described above—heavily cushioned, sloping significantly from heel to toe—became widely available only at the end of the 1970s. Because pronation—how much your foot rolls in as you move from landing to toe-off—could be easily measured in labs, shoe companies made controlling pronation one of the guiding paradigms for designing shoes.

But the primary elements of conventional running shoe design were never proven to be meaningful before they were foisted on millions of runners. "Not every injury is related to pronation and overpronation," says Brian Fullem, a sport podiatrist with 3 decades of running experience and a 14:25 5-K PR. "You need a certain amount of pronation to help absorb shock. And the heel height, I don't know where that came from. The running shoe industry had a 12-millimeter heel-to-toe drop as standard, and there was never any basis for that."

By the end of last decade, this rejection of conventional running shoes was no longer confined to a small group of longtime competitive runners. Nike had introduced the Free, which it marketed as a "training tool" to help strengthen the feet and lower legs. Christopher McDougall's *Born to Run* became an unlikely bestseller and introduced minimalism to the masses. Research suggesting that modern running shoes contributed to poor form and increased risk of injury got mainstream press. Some runners, like Mark Tomkinson, found their running reborn and spoke of the switch to minimalism in evangelical terms. But many more runners, like Mimi Englander, discovered that simply switching shoes wasn't a cure-all and could lead to problems of its own.

As more runners started running in less shoe, blogs and message boards filled with vigorous, often rancorous debate on the topic. As often happens with suddenly hot topics, people at the extremes were the loudest and most involved in the debate, regardless of their level of knowledge. People often universalized from their experience and shouted past each other. The terms of the discussion got oversimplified: Is barefoot running good? Should you throw away your old running shoes? Aren't those people prancing around in those toe shoes going to wreck their feet?

About This Book

Meanwhile, most runners read and heard about barefoot running and minimalism, and kept right on doing whatever they'd always done. After all, minimalist shoes accounting for 11 percent of running shoe sales means that conventional running shoes account for 89 percent of running shoe sales.

This book is for those runners, the vast majority of whom are curious about minimalism and barefoot running but still have some basic questions: Why is changing from conventional shoes worth considering? What is the most relevant information on the topic? How can I experiment with minimalism in a safe, sustainable way that will improve my running?

I've organized this book to answer these questions in a logical way. Before we get started on the specifics, I want to give you an idea where I'm coming from.

The basic premise of this book is that minimalism and barefoot running are means to an end. That end is running with better form and less injury, both of which should make you faster and help you enjoy your running more.

It's important to keep this means-to-an-end framework in mind. Minimalism and barefoot running are tools, not magic bullets. As Jay Johnson, who has coached national champions, collegiate runners, and recreational runners, says, "I think most people want the easy fix. There's no easy answer in running. Ever!"

That's another way of saying that, in running, there are no secrets—either of modern elites or of supposedly lost tribes. There are, however, best practices worked out through experimentation by ambitious, experienced, open-minded runners. The distinction matters because secrets imply, "Do this one thing and everything will be fixed." Best practices imply, "Here's a process that you can implement to improve as a runner."

"There are no secrets" also means keeping the importance of this or any aspect of running in perspective. There's no one element of running that deserves obsessive focus while you underemphasize other contributors to successful running. What you have on your feet when you run matters a lot. So do a lot of other things: how much and how far you run, how strong and flexible you are, your diet, your running form, and how you spend your nonrunning time. Zealotry never works out over the long term in running.

Throughout this book, our conceptual framework will be a model that former Nike Oregon Project coach Steve Magness, a real student of the sport, uses to judge the merits of ideas. He calls it the three legs of the stool, with the legs being theory, research, and practical. "If you have all three legs of the stool aligned, then you can be pretty sure an idea is legit," Magness says. "If you have two legs of the stool, you can sometimes make it work, depending on how strong those two legs are. If you have just one solid leg, then it's obviously not going to stand."

In running terms, the practical leg of the stool most often means looking at what the most successful runners have been doing over the longest period of time. Elite runners aren't a different species from the rest of us. Yes, they have more genetic running aptitude than most people. But they do the same sport we all do; like everyone, they're subject to gravity and apathy. Through unfathomable hours of practice and thought, their trial-and-error process reveals what works best most of the time for most runners. The same is true of runners who've been consistently able to meet their goals over long stretches of time. They have things to teach other runners.

That's why the experts we'll hear from in this book are for the most part not the ones usually cited when you read about minimalism. Our guides will be running experts with deep knowledge and experience throughout the sport, not just in minimalism. They're best able to place minimalism in perspective and show how it fits in with other aspects of long-term healthy and happy running.

In most chapters, we'll also meet runners who describe themselves as minimalists. My goal in presenting these "Meet a Minimalist" profiles is to highlight the range of discoveries—and mistakes—runners often make when they start experimenting with running in less shoe. In some cases, the experiment seems to have gone well; in other cases, not so well. Read the profiles to learn ordinary runners' experiences with minimalism, while bearing in mind that there are many variables that affect success and failure in running. That is, read the profiles more to gather general ideas than to find models to mimic.

A NOTE FROM THE AUTHOR

I've run more than 100,000 miles since I started running as a teen-ager in 1979. I've run almost all those miles in light, low-to-the-ground shoes. At first that was because such shoes were pretty much all that was available. But even after more cushioned shoes became the norm, I instinctively gravitated toward the light, low models. They just made running more enjoyable. When I ran in bulkier models—most often while testing them for magazine shoe reviews—I spent most of the run noticing the shoes—how they felt too heavy, how I felt suspended off the ground and tilted forward by the large heel.

I began barefoot running not long after I started the sport. In 10th grade my running geek friends and I read advice from coaches in *Runner's World, Running Times,* and *The Runner* (now defunct). They recommended small amounts of barefoot running to strengthen the feet and improve form. And we knew our history— how Abebe Bikila won the 1960 Olympic Marathon barefoot and how world-class Europeans sometimes raced on the track barefoot. On most easy days, our coach had us do 10 100-meter strides on grass. My friends and I started doing these sessions barefoot. We loved how the grass felt under our feet, and we had that eager-teen belief that we were training smarter than our rivals.

As it turned out, my school district didn't allow athletes to leave school grounds for practice. So instead of hitting the roads on days we weren't working out on the track, we were confined to a 1-mile perimeter of the school. It was almost entirely grass. Around and around and around we'd go, 5, 8, 10 times. This was also where we warmed up and cooled down on track days. My friends and I enjoyed our barefoot striders so much that we started doing our cooldowns barefoot. That felt good. We started doing some regular runs on easy days barefoot. That felt good, too. One Saturday I drove to school and did a barefoot 14-miler on that perimeter loop. It remains one of the most enjoyably memorable solo runs of my life.

The point of all this is that I've been what would now be called a minimalist my entire running life. Long before I started thinking about writing a book on minimalism, I watched the movement's evolution with great interest. In the early part of this century, I was the kook. Friends would see me doing regular runs in racing shoes and ask, "How can you run in those?" I'd point at the huge midsoles and heels of their shoes and ask, "How can you run in those?" When they'd say something like, "I like the cushioning," I'd respond, "Why that amount? Why not twice as much, or three times as much?" They would just shrug and we'd get on with our run. Like I said, I was the kook.

By the end of the decade, I was the boring old fart. Acquaintances would tell stories of reading *Born to Run*, switching immediately from their conventional running shoes to a barely there model, or even starting to run in Vibram FiveFingers after years of inactivity, and finding themselves injured. "Shocking," I'd say in my unhelpful way. Casual runners—even nonrunners like my in-laws—would ask, "What do you think about barefoot running?" and I'd either give an answer far more long and involved than they wanted, full of caveats and codicils, or just sigh and try to change the topic.

Of course, all that time, my opinion and practices were more or less unchanged: Running in as little shoe as you can while staying a healthy, happy runner is a good goal. This isn't a new development in running, a secret, or a magic bullet. It's simply a goal that may help you enjoy your running more. And really, what more do any of us want from our running than to enjoy it on our terms for the rest of our lives?

To work toward that goal, use the same slow-burn ambition that the late Grete Waitz, nine-time winner of the New York City Marathon, advised for success in any area of running. "Hurry slowly," Waitz said. "Be dedicated and disciplined and work hard, but take your time. Move ahead, but be patient."

The first step toward meeting any goal is understanding why it's worthwhile. Let's start by looking at the most basic question about minimalism: Why bother?

CHAPTER 2

WHY BOTHER?

Reasons for running in less shoe

THE FOCUS ON MINIMALIST FOOTWEAR sometimes obscures an important point: Running in lighter, lower, flatter shoes (or no shoes) isn't an end goal, but a means to an end. That end is a more efficient, more effective running gait. Better running form should translate to increased performance, decreased risk of injury, and, harder to quantify but still important, greater enjoyment of your running. (Who wouldn't like to feel more fluid and flowing on their runs?) Many runners who've successfully transitioned to running in minimalist shoes—by which I mean they're running the mileage they want largely injury-free—report achieving these benefits.

These are compelling reasons to consider running in minimalist shoes. Anything you can do to lower your risk of injury should translate to increased performance, in that you'll be able to accumulate long stretches of consistent training. If there's one thing that running experts agree on, it's that consistency is key to running your best.

As always in running, there are caveats. Yes, running in minimalist shoes can help change your form for the better. And yes, running with good form is better than running with poorer form. But there's more to running than your form. There's mileage and hard workouts, strength and flexibility, diet and attitude, and many other contributors to success.

For too long, the majority of non-elite runners barely thought about their form. Now the pendulum has quickly swung to the other extreme, and form has become an obsession for some runners. They ask: Should I switch to a midfoot strike? Should I increase my cadence? Should I run upright or with a forward lean? How should I hold my thumbs? It's easy to find runners who spend more time online discussing running form than they do running.

Later in this chapter we'll get experts' thoughts on the benefits of minimalist shoes. But first, let's take a step back and get a better understanding of what you should know about running form, no matter what's on your feet.

DON'T JUST RUN, BABY

When Bill Rodgers was the best marathoner in the world in the late 1970s, a biomechanist named Peter Cavanagh tested him in his lab at Penn State. As part of the test, Cavanagh had Rodgers "fix" his trademark across-the-body right arm swing. The result? Running with more textbook form, Rodgers consumed more oxygen at the same pace. That is, changing Rodgers's form to something thought to be better made it more "costly" for him to run a given pace; what's known as his running economy worsened.

In the 3½ decades since that lab experiment, a take-home message from it has been endlessly repeated: Don't mess with your running form. Over time, your body will find its best way of running. The more you run, the more your body will find its natural form. Just run, baby.

Why, then, do almost all top coaches have their runners spend time working on their form? Why do most elites, already blessed with enviable technique, think that working on their form will make them faster, either directly or by allowing them to train more by avoiding injury? And why should you?

For starters, let's go back to the Rodgers experiment. No reputable source claims that, at any one instant, significantly altering your form from what your body is used to will make you faster. Coaching legend and longtime exercise-science lab rat Jack Daniels, PhD, has tested thousands of runners over the last 40 years. "I have tested runners' economy of running with their hands in their pockets, on their hips, folded on top of their heads, etc., and it always costs more than when using a normal arm swing," he says.

But that doesn't mean the logical conclusion is that the form your body naturally gravitates toward is what will make you fastest. "We all run as children and assume that we are doing it correctly," says two-time Olympic marathoner Pete Pfitzinger, now general manager of capacity and expertise at High Performance Sport NZ in New Zealand. "That is usually not a bad assumption, but there is a difference between doing something reasonably well and maximizing performance." Pfitzinger says that many runners can improve their running economy—again, their oxygen cost at a given pace—by 2 to 4 percent through improved form. "If you have been training hard for several years, it can be an easier way to improve than doing more repeat miles."

Nor does it mean that your "natural" form is in your best long-term interest. "When we go out and run, we have a pattern of form that follows our skeleton and is dictated by our muscles and range of motion," says veteran coach Roy Benson, who has worked with high schoolers, Olympians, beginners, and everyone in between. "Over the course of lots of running, it's like an electrical current—your body follows the path of least resistance."

Running with "least resistance" sounds great, right? Doesn't this mean you're running as efficiently as possible?

Not necessarily. Pete Magill, who holds several American age-group records and has coached runners for more than 2 decades, says, "This belief system that just doing it over and over is somehow going to make us better is really crazy. Longtime runners actually suffer from the body's ability to become efficient. You become so efficient that you start recruiting fewer muscle fibers to do the same exercise, and as you begin using fewer muscle fibers, you start to get a little bit weaker. Over time, that can become significant. Once you've stopped recruiting as many fibers, you start exerting too much pressure on the fibers you are recruiting to perform the same action. And then you start getting muscle imbalance injuries—calf strains, little hamstring pulls, things like that."

Magill adds, with more than a little frustration in his voice, "Running is the one sport where people think, 'I don't have to worry about my technique. I'm not carrying a ball, I'm not swinging a bat, I'm not on skates, so my form doesn't matter.' We also have a sport where people don't always listen to what the top people are doing. They're far more interested in what the local Pose guru (see "Form Schools" on page 19) might be telling them than in what [two-time Olympic marathoner] Ryan Hall is doing. I would say all top runners work to improve their form."

Certainly that's been my observation. In the past 2 decades, professional responsibilities have given me the privilege of observing the training of scores of runners. I've seen every top runner I've spent more than a little time around work on form, either directly through technique drills, indirectly through strengthening work, or simply by being mindful of form while running.

What's Good Running Form?

It's important when discussing running form to remember that there's no "perfect" form that we should all aspire to. And, adds Pfitzinger, "No one can look at you and say whether your running economy is good or bad. We would all try to 'fix' Paula Radcliffe if classic running technique was synonymous with good running economy." That's Pfitzinger's nice way of saying that the women's marathon world record holder can be tiring just to watch running, given how her head bobs and weaves like she's in a sparring match. And yet looks often deceive when it comes to running form. In one experiment, Daniels tested a group's running economy, then showed footage of the runners to coaches and had them rank who, based on running form, had the best running economy. The coaches' answers were no more accurate than if they had guessed randomly.

So how to know if you should bother working on your form? And again, why do elites spend time doing so?

University of Illinois coach Jeremy Rasmussen puts it this way: "I bet that if I went out and said we're going to do functional testing on a sample of people, you're going to find weaknesses in every single one of them. The body has adapted to who you are, but has the body adapted to the best possible thing you can offer it? No, because you have inefficiencies somewhere, so if you can change those inefficiencies and make them strengths, then your body will start to change naturally for the better." Rasmussen works on form with all his runners, including three-time NCAA champion Angela Bizzarri, who won those championships and overcame a history of injury only after she and Rasmussen worked to improve how she covers the ground.

Magill agrees, especially for the many over-40 runners he works with. "I assume that any runner who's been away from youthful activities like basketball, Frisbee, football, tennis—been away from a wide variety of activities that actually work on muscle balance—I assume that they haven't been trained for a full range of motion and that they've developed muscle imbalances."

FORM SCHOOLS

Various prescriptions for running form have become popular in recent years. ChiRunning and the Pose Method are the best known.

These methods have much good to say about running form, including working toward a lighter, quicker cadence and avoiding heavy heel-striking. Where the vast majority of successful coaches and runners find fault with the schools is the idea that there's one precise, perfect way to run that's universally applicable. Most also question the near-myopic emphasis on form, rather than considering it one of several elements of peak performance. And, it's fair to ask,

where are all the world-class runners who follow these methods to a T?

Many non-elite runners have found their running invigorated and improved by ChiRunning and the Pose Method. This isn't surprising, in the same way that people who go on a diet often lose weight, regardless of whether it's high-carb or low-carb, gluten-free or grain-heavy. Simply paying attention to what they're eating is enough of a change from their normal habits for many people to lose weight. Similarly, working on their form is different enough from many runners' past practices to cause significant improvements.

While there's no perfect form, there are common elements of good form, based on basic principles of physics and biomechanics. These include:

Footstrike. A true forefoot landing is rare and can be as inefficient as a heavy heel landing. Somewhere between a slight heel landing and midfoot is best for most people. A midfoot landing allows release at toe-off of energy stored in your calf muscles and Achilles tendons. Over time, your footstrike should move toward what's natural for you if you're running in shoes that don't negatively change your gait and if you have proper strength.

Landing position. Make ground contact near your body's center of mass, with your landing knee slightly bent and your lower leg close to perpendicular to the ground.

Midflight. When both feet are off the ground, you still want to be traveling forward more than you are vertically. Too much vertical motion (for example, if you see the horizon bobbing up and down) means you're wasting energy to go in a different direction than you want to be.

Knee lift. Your amount of knee lift should be in sync with how fast you're going, from almost none when you're jogging easily, on up to your thigh being parallel to the ground when you're close to

BORN TO HEEL-STRIKE?

Coach Steve Magness says that runners are heel-strikers for different reasons. Here's how he distinguishes them.

"I have someone who's a heavy heel-striker do strides with their shoes on, then have them take their shoes off and do strides," Magness says. "If they still heel-strike barefoot, then you know it's a motor programming thing, because it's not the weight of the shoe or heel-toe drop or feedback blocked by the shoe. So then it's, 'All right, this is how this person tends to run.' Then you have to take an approach of 'We've got to do some actual mechanical work and give some cues and try to consciously change things.'

"If that's not the case, then I think you go the other route and adjust the surroundings via strengthening work, shoe choice, and dynamic flexibility."

sprinting, and with an appropriate increase as you move from your slowest pace to your fastest pace.

Turnover. There's no magic number of strides per minutes that's universally desirable, but most people will run most efficiently at a cadence of 170 to 180 steps per minute (that is, each foot striking the ground 85 to 90 times per minute). Your turnover should increase somewhat the faster you're going, but that 170-to-180 range is appropriate for most of your runs. When I did some easy runs in Kenya with guys who'd run under 13:00 for 5-K, their turnover was the same as when they got rolling.

Upper body. Run straight with a slight forward lean (which is different from bent over at the waist). Your arms should be at 90 degrees, your shoulders low and level, your hands held loosely cupped, neither in tight fists nor flopping around. Swing your arms up from the hip, not out, and try to keep them from crossing your body laterally. The insides of your wrists should come near your waist as your arms come through.

What deviations from this basic model do experts most often see?

Daniels says that in young and old runners alike he's worked with, "The most common form problem was stride rate—bounding over the ground too slowly, with long strides. Runners are often told to work on a long stride, but that is more a function of getting fitter rather than just doing it. I never had a runner perform worse when I felt they needed a faster rhythm and they learned to use a faster cadence." Minimalist shoes help many runners develop this quicker cadence.

Benson and Pfitzinger also see more overstriding than they would like. Says Pfitzinger, "My observation of runners in road races is that hardly any of the elite runners overstride, but up to

20 percent of the runners slower than 40:00 for 10-K overstride. Increasing stride rate by a few percent and decreasing stride length by a few percent can improve running economy in most overstriders." Here, too, minimalist shoes are often helpful.

Pfitzinger says other form problems he often sees include:

- Leaning forward at the waist, which causes the quads to work harder to keep you from falling forward.

ARE YOU OVERSTRIDING?

There's a difference between overstriding and having a long stride. Overstriding means that your feet land significantly in front of your center of mass. When this happens, you're unable to make full use of your fitness, because you're braking with every step. And you might soon be breaking with every step, in that overstriding amplifies the already-strong impact forces of running and therefore can contribute to more strain on your bones, muscles, and ligaments.

Veteran coach Roy Benson suggests these two methods of determining if you're overstriding:

First, have a friend with a video camera stand 20 yards back from the side of a level surface. Run past your friend for 30 to 40 yards at an easy pace. Then run past the camera at around 10-K race pace. Finally, run at a near sprint.

Says Benson, "When you watch yourself, even though you might not be able to stop action and analyze it at that level, just by seeing your form you can recognize whether you're overstriding. As long as your knee is bent and your foot is coming down back underneath you or close to you, there's probably not much

- Obviously not using the glute muscles. "When the glutes aren't working, the leg typically does not straighten behind the body, so the stride is more in front and under the body than behind the body," says Pfitzinger. "It looks like the runner is running just with the quads and hamstrings. Often the calves also don't do much, because they are the last push at the back of the stride. There is very little push behind the body, and the stride is relatively short."

inefficiency and not much risk."

Second, have a friend stand in front of you while you run toward her at the three effort levels in the above exercise. Says Benson, "The friend looks to see how much of the sole of your shoe is showing on impact. If there's 4, 5, 6 inches of daylight between your toe and the ground when your heel hits, you're overstriding."

The three effort levels are important, Benson explains, because many runners, especially those who didn't compete in school, become overstriders only when they try to go faster.

To improve a tendency to overstride, practice running fast while landing over your center of mass.

This is often best done by going to a field or other safe, soft surface and shedding your shoes.

Says Benson, "At first, jog in place. You'll be landing on the ball of your foot. That's what it feels like to be a midfoot-striker. Now stay up there and jog in place and lean over and slowly accelerate over the next 50 yards or so. Don't go so fast that you forget to stay up there and land on the ball of your foot. When you do them right, strides like these are fast enough to be a good way to teach midfoot-striking." Then stay conscious of what that footstrike feels like, especially when you do track workouts and other faster sessions.

- Holding the head forward of the center of gravity, which makes the neck and upper-back muscles fire to keep the head from falling forward.

Magill says, for longtime runners, "I assume you're not getting the same knee lift you used to get. Even for people who do tempo runs

DON'T FORCE FORM CHANGES

If your car is out of alignment, you can keep driving it by continually jerking it in a direction it doesn't want to go, or you can get the alignment fixed.

If you want to significantly change an aspect of your running form, such as switching from a heel to midfoot landing, don't take the jerking-the-steering-wheel approach. "I'm not a real fan of contrived changes," says physiotherapist and 2:23 marathoner Phil Wharton. "They're not sustainable—the body will just keep reverting if you don't have the necessary flexibility and strength. Or, neurologically you're not yet ready to change that movement pattern. I feel like so many people are jumping ahead to the foot placement or some other isolated part of their form before they have the functioning body to sustain it. Get the functioning, and then the form will just start to naturally come."

There's a difference between being mindful of the elements of good form and forcing your body to run in a way it's not yet ready to. All good training is a gradual accumulation of small gains. Be diligent about monitoring your form to correct less-than-ideal habits. But also be diligent about strengthening and other work that will improve your running body and enable you to run naturally with better form.

and reps, they rarely run faster than the race pace they're expecting to go. Let's say your shortest distance is 5-K and you almost never regularly run faster than 5-K race pace. Well, if that's 100 percent of what you're training your body to do, then it's a 100 percent effort for your body to lift your knees to the level you have to at 5-K race pace. Your body's going to find it's easier to hit 90 percent of that max effort, and you're not going to get the knee lift you need to run as fast as you want, and that's just going to compound over time."

FORM FIXES

There's more to improving your running form than switching shoes. Some people can run with poor form barefoot; others can have exquisite mechanics in moon boots. That being the case, if you want to improve your form, there are things to address beyond footwear.

First, become an overall better athlete through regular short bouts of running at faster than race pace, strengthening your core and other key body parts, and by performing form drills. Says Magill, "If you can strengthen your muscles so that you can move strongly through a fuller range of motion, you can take the fitness you already have and run faster." Benson agrees, saying, "As you get general strength, you get better form."

If you're thinking, "That's all well and good for college runners and pros, who can train all day, but I have only an hour a day total for my running, so I'm better off spending that time just getting in the miles," Magill has an answer for you.

"That would be a great argument," he says, "if it were true. But if you have only an hour a day to devote to your running, the first thing you've got to do is learn to run. If you bring bad form into your running, all you're going to be doing for that hour a day is reinforcing bad form. If you spent even 1 of those days per week, or just a bit of time in those sessions, now you would be spending time actually training with good form. You'd then be using that hour every day to train with the form that's going to apply to your race speed and to your efficiency when running.

"A lot of people waste far more time being injured from running with muscle imbalances and poorly developed form than they do spending time doing drills or exercises or short hills or setting aside a short period each week to work on form itself."

We'll look at drills and targeted strengthening in Chapter 8.

A second way to have better running form is to minimize the deleterious effects of your nonrunning life. Spending hours a day slumped over in front of a computer wreaks havoc on everyone's body, but especially on a runner's body. Excessive sitting, even with the best posture, shuts off muscle activity along the back of your body; physiotherapist Phil Wharton calls this "glutes in hibernation." These are the very muscles you need to use to run with good form. In addition, the posture most of us adopt when working, texting, driving, and watching TV throws off our body's alignment. In Chapter 8 we'll see how to deal with these potential vectors of inefficiency and injury.

Third, you can work on improving specific parts of your form while running. Rasmussen does much of his form-improvement work by giving runners cues ("fast feet," "shoulders low," etc.) while they do "striders." Throughout this book you'll hear experts recommend striders. These are runs of 60 to 100 meters, done at about the pace you could hold in a mile race. Striders (or "strides" or "strideouts") are done on flat, level ground. The key is to run fast but relaxed—mile race pace, not sprinting. Doing striders once or twice a week after an easy run is a fun, easy way to improve many aspects of your running, including your form. If there's one type of fast running that all runners should do, even runners who never intend to race, it's striders.

Rasmussen also advises short bits of form work on regular runs. "When you go out for your run, for part of your run, pick a light pole that's about 100 meters out," he says. "Pick an aspect of form you want to improve. Focus on that one particular thing for that period of time, and then go back to just running, and then a few minutes later find another light pole and do it again, and bring it into your normal runs that way. Over time you can feel the difference."

Finally, when this all starts to seem too much to worry about for what's a basic human motion, relax. Literally. Says Daniels, "While running, go over your body from head to toe and ask yourself: 'Am I relaxed in the eyes? Am I relaxed in the jaw? Am I relaxed in the neck and shoulders? Am I relaxed in the arms and hands? Am I relaxed in the hips, in the knees, in the ankles, in the feet?' You may find some tight areas that may lead to better economy if fixed."

THE BEEF WITH BEEFY SHOES

Now we can circle back to shoes. If you had to give the 30-second pro-minimalism pitch, it would be some version of this:

Because of their high heels and plush cushioning, conventional running shoes alter many elements of good running form. They encourage runners to run differently than if they were running barefoot—in big shoes, runners tend to land hard on their heels, to overstride, and to lose valuable feedback that comes from "feeling" the ground. These changes can lead to less efficient running, eventual injury, and gradual weakening of the feet and lower limbs. The onus is on conventional shoes, not minimalist shoes, to prove their value, because minimalist shoes encourage and allow more natural running form while providing necessary protection from surface hazards.

Experts from throughout running agree with this argument.

"I definitely think that some people benefit from the minimalist shoes," says sport podiatrist Brian Fullem. "Especially if they're able to change their stride and get off their heels, that may help eliminate some running pains people have in their knees, or shin splints or other injuries that may be increased by landing on your heels."

"Midfoot is the best place to land, and obviously if the shoe has too much in the rear, your propensity is to land more toward the back of the foot," says Wharton. "My clinical experience over the last 24 years is that people's feet get weaker by wearing high heels, by wearing shoes that don't fit properly, by having too narrow a toe-box. There are all kinds of conditions that come from the wrong shoes—you get hammertoe, you get hallux valgus, where the big toe comes in. And that's one of the most important joints to have working, to get up on your metatarsals to propel yourself properly when walking or running."

Wharton's comments here touch on another common minimalist-versus-conventional-shoe design difference, in that minimalist shoes tend to be constructed to allow the foot to work naturally. That includes a wide toebox to allow the toes to splay as you roll through the gait cycle. Most traditional running shoes restrict this movement because they taper from the ball of the foot to the front of the shoe.

Referring to the three-legged-stool means of weighing scientific evidence discussed in Chapter 1, coach Steve Magness says, "If you look at the theory leg of the stool, you have some good theory—that conventional training shoes change mechanics and might block feedback, and that minimalist shoes can help strengthen you and let you better utilize elastic energy."

In Chapter 4, we'll look in depth at another leg of that stool—research—and see exactly what the data show on how people run differently when shod or barefoot, as well as what the research says about injury rates and running economy in different types of footwear. For now, it's enough to acknowledge that most runners run differently when they switch from conventional running shoes to barely there models. Just ask the calves of someone who immediately runs for an hour in Vibram FiveFingers after years in conventional shoes.

"One of the main effects of going to the more minimalist footwear is that it pretty much forces you to shorten your stride a bit," says minimalist blogger and college biology professor Peter Larson. "That's the quick fix that changing shoes can bring, and I think that's why some people may see an almost immediate result by changing shoes, because it forces you to change your stride in certain ways."

It's worth reemphasizing that this is a change for the better. It's a change toward a more natural running form, the form you would use barefoot and if you didn't have years of bad habits ingrained in your muscle memory.

MEET A MINIMALIST

CAMILLE HERRON
WARR ACRES, OKLAHOMA

Camille Herron is the rare national-class marathoner who's a full-blown minimalist. She credits ditching orthotics and conventional running shoes with allowing her to overcome a history of stress fractures, run prodigious mileage, lower her marathon PR to 2:37, and, to top it off, frequently win marathons.

After suffering her third stress fracture in her left foot as a high school runner, Herron was given orthotics and told to wear them with traditional trainers. Four more stress fractures prevented her from seriously competing in college. She became, in her words, "a hobby jogger."

At the same time, Herron's physics, biomechanics, and kinesiology classes got her thinking about the basics of the running gait. She also read stories of Kenyans running long distances barefoot. After yet another injury in the fall of 2003, she'd had enough—she committed to starting from scratch and rebuilding herself as a minimalist runner years before most runners had heard of the concept.

"I decided to go cold turkey and ditch my orthotics and the shoes I'd been training in," she says. "I think the first run I tried to do was in house slippers. I thought, 'Yeah, that might be a little too minimal,' so I ended up getting a pair of retro Asics flats."

Frustrated by so many years of setbacks, Herron had the patience to progress slowly. She started by running 2 or 3 miles every other day. In her first month, she hit 10 miles a week. In her second month, 20 miles a week. She added 10 miles per week each month, and by June 2004, at age 22, she was running 70 miles a week injury-free.

But not necessarily ache-free, at least at first. "During the first few months, I had very sore ankles and calves," Herron says. "My arches were pretty sore, too, but it was the kind of soreness or stiffness that felt okay, like the kind you might get with any new training program. I'd hobble out of bed in the morning wondering when my feet were going to stop bothering me. Then one day in March 2004, I woke up and got out of bed and I felt fine."

Herron also started experimenting with barefoot running at this time. Here, too, she took a gradual approach—5 minutes at a time, then 10 minutes, then up to 20 to 30 minutes a few times a week, on grass, within a few months. She ran barefoot as therapy when her legs felt tired or, her word, quirky. "If my Achilles would feel tweaked or my plantar felt off, I'd do some barefoot running, and it felt like it healed my body," she says.

These days, she still does some barefoot running, weather permitting, but mostly in the form of strides and drills. Herron is sponsored by inov-8 and says, "The inov-8s have more of a minimal build than the shoes I wore when I was sponsored by Brooks, so I feel like I haven't had to do any barefoot running to reset my body like I used to."

Herron consistently runs 120 to 140 miles a week in the inov-8 230s or 233s after initially trying slighter inov-8 models, the 155s and 195s. "It's interesting, I've gone from less shoe to a little more shoe," she says. "I think it's a matter of over time for the marathon you need a little bit more cushion-ing because you're spending more time on your feet."

In 2011, Herron did indeed spend a lot of time on her feet—she wound up with just under 6,000 miles for the year. That included running six marathons, and winning three of them. Does she therefore think everyone should take her approach?

"I don't know if other people can do what I did and be successful with it, but it's something to try if all else fails," she says. "If someone feels like they're okay, I would stick with what works. The key is to be healthy and to be able to train consistently, regardless of what's on your feet. Definitely if you keep getting hurt, it could be your shoes, especially if you have a lot of foot injuries, Achilles problems, plantar problems."

For herself, though, she's sold. "To have gone from seven stress fractures to no stress fractures and being able to handle high mileage," Herron says, "it definitely says something about how it's changed my gait, made me stop overstriding, and changed the stresses on my feet and lower legs."

Minimalist shoes can help bring about another positive change—reviving your feet's ability to work to their full mechanical potential. That can occur in two ways. First, you can improve your proprioceptive ability, which is sensing what's underfoot and making minute, instant changes to adapt optimally to changes in terrain. Second, your feet can relearn how to change from a flexible platform when you land to a rigid propulsive lever as you toe off. These mechanical gains can help increase efficiency, lower your risk of injury, and just make running feel better.

Embracing minimalism is also a healthy change in mind-set—to emphasizing that running is a natural, healthy activity, rather than something we dare to do only in "protective" and "supportive" shoes.

WHERE ARE ALL THE ELITE MINIMALISTS?

Runners who are skeptical about minimalism often ask a simple question: If minimalism leads to better form and performance and fewer injuries, why do the best runners in the world do a lot of their mileage in conventional shoes? Even if full-on minimalism caused only a fraction of a percentage of improvement, shouldn't the people whose races are decided by hundredths of a second be among its greatest adherents? Given everything else that elites do to get even the slightest edge, why not this?

These are fair questions that merit an in-depth answer. To start, let's make clear that we're not talking here about trail ultramarathoners or other excellent niche runners, but the sort who contend for Olympic teams and national titles. That is, the best at the type of running that most competitive runners do.

The observation that there are few world-class full-time minimalists is accurate. Elite runners run a lot in conventional running shoes. This is true not just in the United States, where today's stars grew up as conventionally shod young runners. I once spent a month in Iten, Kenya, a small town on the edge of the Rift Valley that's the epicenter of Kenyan running. Nary a minimalist was in sight. Kenyans may grow up barefoot, but once they have access to conventional running shoes, they wear them. A few years ago, one of the organizations that provide donated running shoes to needy Kenyan runners was given 300 pairs of Vibram FiveFingers to distribute. None of the Kenyans wanted them.

There are a few key points to consider in unraveling why most elites aren't minimalists:

If minimalist shoes are a means to an end, most elites already have attained that end. That is, almost all elites have the form that non-elites running in minimalist shoes aspire to. One reason they've been above-average runners since their first step is because their bodies are inherently better at running efficiently.

"For the most part they're already very biomechanically sound," says Wharton. "They're already landing up front, in the mid- to forefoot, so they don't really need to do everything in minimalist shoes to help them get there. You look at [world champion and Olympic medalist] Bernard Lagat and it's hard to see anything you'd want to change." Also, remember from earlier in this chapter that almost all elites do regular form work, another means toward this end.

For elites, the potential payoff in slight form improvement isn't worth the risk. That risk comes in two forms—injury from a too-rapid transition and reduced mileage and/or intensity while transitioning. "Out of 52 weeks a year, the average elite is healthy maybe 48 weeks a year," says Jay Johnson, who's coached runners to national titles in cross-country and indoor track. "They're going to say, 'I could potentially lose a lot of training getting used to doing all my running in these flimsy little shoes, and I don't know that it's going to make me any better.'"

Magness, who used to work with double Olympic gold medalist Mo Farah and Olympic silver medalist Galen Rupp, says, "The bang for the buck isn't there. If you can train in a mixture of shoes and be injury-free, then why make any sort of transition? That's why the few elites and sub-elites who you see do all their training in minimalist shoes are the ones who don't have anything to lose. They were always injured, and they were like, 'This is a last-ditch effort. It's worth a shot.'"

Cushioning has its merits. Running easily, for as much or as little as you feel like doing on any given day, is a natural activity. But training to be the best in the world is extraordinarily hard. It places varied demands on the body. World-class runners require different solutions—and different shoes—depending on their training.

"Sometimes the smartest thing to do with shoes is to match the shoe to fatigue level," says Magness. "If Galen Rupp has just done a long track workout in spikes and his calves are completely beat up, then they're not going to do any of the cushioning job they normally do. So you throw on some heavy, padded trainers and let the legs recover."

Elites have always done a lot of running in minimalist shoes. They just don't call them "minimalist shoes." They call them spikes and racing flats and lightweight trainers, and they wear them for almost all their hard workouts. Someone like Rupp might run 30 or 40 miles a week in light, low-to-the-ground shoes, the same amount as many minimalists' weekly mileage. ("And with a heck of a lot more force!" Johnson points out.) It's just that Rupp runs another 70 to 80 miles on top of that.

"That's the crux of this," says Magness. "Elites spend a lot of time in flats and spikes and lightweight trainers. And they'll do some easy barefoot mileage. I think most coaches agree that's going to get us all the bang for our buck in terms of performance enhancement or injury prevention or mechanics changes. Are we really going to gain from switching to minimalist shoes for the regular easy runs?"

Gold medalist Frank Shorter once told his fellow Olympic marathoner Kenny Moore, "You say you don't believe in high mileage, but you sure as hell run high mileage." Look at what successful runners do, not what arbitrarily defined camp they or others put them in. In the case of minimalism, that means recognizing that elites run a lot of miles in what most people would call minimalist shoes, while acknowledging that they also run a lot of miles in what most people would call conventional running shoes.

As it turns out, there was a time when all elites did all their running in minimalist shoes. In fact, all runners did. A brief survey of running shoe history is in order.

CHAPTER 3

A BRIEF HISTORY OF MINIMALISM

There was a time
when all shoes were minimalist

HERE ARE SOME USER COMMENTS I recently read about a popular New Balance running shoe:

"Flexibility gives feeling of next-to-nothingness," one runner wrote. Another praised the shoe's "ground-hugging feel." Then again, another runner pointed out, the shoe's "soles wear out too fast," "every grain of sand feels like an egg," and they offer "insufficient support."

Hmm, maybe a popular Adidas shoe would be better. It "conforms to the natural shape of the foot," one runner wrote. It "makes you want to run fast," a second commented. But, a third warned, it's "too thin for races as long as a marathon."

I read on, hoping an upstart company's innovative model, designed by a leading coach, might deliver nirvana. It's "made on a last conforming to the natural shape of the foot," one runner wrote, while others said it provides "excellent inside support and balance, good cushioning, plenty of toe room, relief from recurrent foot and leg problems." And yet, despite being one of the most expensive running shoes on the market, its "soles and heels wear too quickly," another runner cautioned.

I read these insights not in the latest *Running Times* shoe review or on a message board, but in a special *Runner's World* "booklet of the month," *All About Distance Running Shoes.*

If the title of the booklet—not to mention the idea of a booklet of the month—sounds a little off, that's probably because said booklet was published in July 1971. The New Balance shoe reviewed was the Jogster ("formerly Trackster II," the booklet informs, but you probably already knew that). The Adidas model was the Marathon. The new kid on the block was the Lydiard Road Runner, developed with input from the legendary New Zealand coach Arthur Lydiard. Perhaps his consulting fee was why the shoe cost $19.95, a dollar more than the Jogster. The most expensive shoe in the booklet was the Puma Marathon, which, at $26, cost more than twice as much as the Tiger Marathon, a steal at $11.95. (Imagine three companies today giving a shoe the same name.)

All About Distance Running Shoes shows that much of minimalism isn't new. For that matter, in the 4 decades since its publication, not much has changed in runners' attitudes toward shoes. One runner quoted in the booklet noted, "Each time a shoe comes along, I eagerly anticipate the wearing of them and hope they solve my problems. I am always disappointed." Another put it this way: "Light shoes are nice, but my feet get awful sore in a long race, and thus reduces my morale and 'fight' badly sometimes. Heavy shoes reduce the amount of foot pain but increase leg fatigue. You can't win."

It's worth learning a bit about running shoes of old, for fun and context. Whether the topic is training or diet, gadgets or gear, being a student of the sport helps to provide perspective when weighing others' statements about running.

MINIMALISM AS THE DEFAULT

In *All About Distance Running Shoes*, the Tiger Cortez was praised for its "high heel" and being "effective for absorbing shock on hard pavement." The shoe "feels like running on pillows," one runner gushed. Not so fast, others countered; the Cortez was "too mushy" and "feels like a logging boot."

That reads like what today's runners might say, good and bad, about current conventional shoes. The Cortez is the anomaly in the booklet. The rest of the road running shoes look like what today would be classified as minimalist models—low to the ground, a simple upper and outsole construction, little or no difference in heel height and forefoot height. One big difference: Because of

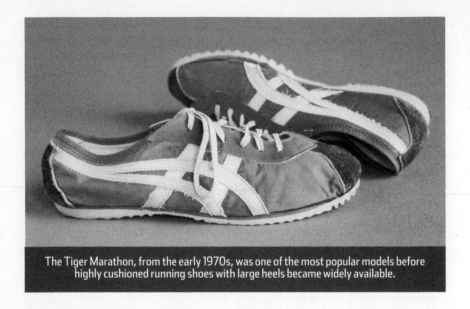

The Tiger Marathon, from the early 1970s, was one of the most popular models before highly cushioned running shoes with large heels became widely available.

manufacturing processes and materials of 4 decades ago, many of the models in *All About Distance Running Shoes* are heavy by today's standards. Whereas the current New Balance Minimus Road weighs 6.1 ounces in a men's size 9, the New Balance Jogster of old weighed 11 ounces in a size 8. (One clue about running demographics of that time is that weights for women's sizes aren't listed in the booklet, as there were almost no women runners, and certainly not mass-produced shoes made specifically for women to run in.)

But there were some light shoes. The Adidas Marathon weighed 8.5 ounces in a size 8, in line with many of today's minimalist models. The Tiger Marathon, the booklet informs in an oddly precise detail, weighed 6.24 ounces in a size 8. I measured its heel height at 10 millimeters and forefoot height at 8 millimeters. Compare that with a current shoe like the Vivobarefoot Evo II, which is one of the lowest shoes on the market, with heel and forefoot heights of 7 millimeters. If available today, the Tiger Marathon would appeal as much to minimalist runners as to urban hipsters.

I borrowed *All About Distance Running Shoes* from Dave Kayser, a retired museum curator for the National Park Service who lives in Danvers, Massachusetts. In addition to marbles, advertising pins, and telephone pole insulators (!), Kayser collects old running shoes. He estimates his collection at about 100. For 12 years he had what he calls "a running tree" in his yard—a fence post with thin

WHO WERE THE RUNNERS OF OLD?

The 1971 booklet *All About Distance Running Shoes* included input from *Runner's World* subscribers. About 800 of them, 15 percent of the magazine's circulation at the time, filled out a questionnaire about their shoes, mileage, and injuries. (Another constant in the sport—runners' love for talking about their running to anyone who'll listen.)

The average respondent was 29 years old, stood 5'9", weighed 145 pounds, had been running for more than 5 years, and averaged nearly 50 miles a week. The respon-

dents were overwhelmingly, if not entirely, male. The differences in demographics compared with today's runners are worth tucking away somewhere in your brain.

Injuries were the bane of runners' existence then as now. Using as the definition of injury a condition that required time off from running and that was caused by running, the *Runner's World* readers reported that the most common injuries were "knee damage" (17.9 percent of respondents), Achilles tendinitis (14 percent), and shin splints (10.6 percent).

strips tacked to the ends of branches that he attached shoes to. (These days Kayser keeps the shoes in his basement.) The earliest mass-production model he owns is the New Balance Trackster, from the 1960s. The oldest models in his collection are spikes from the 1930s and a pair of road shoes from the 1940s, "with kind of a gum sole," he says.

Kayser has been a runner for more than 45 years, with PRs of 53:19 for 10 miles and 2:30 for the marathon. "When I started running, you didn't have much of a selection," he says. "You took what was foisted on you and hoped for the best. Almost all the shoes were low-profile, what today I guess would be called minimalist shoes. That's what almost everyone ran in."

Kayser is bemused by the trends he's seen in shoe preference, as runners rejected the shoes of his youth for heavily cushioned models that were marketed as runners' saviors. "What happened to all the science that was supposedly put into running shoes?" he asks.

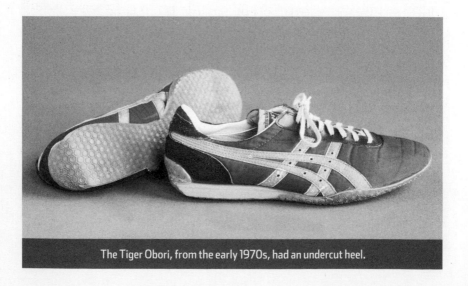

The Tiger Obori, from the early 1970s, had an undercut heel.

"Over the years they'd say, 'Oh, this is the greatest shoe because our studies show blah, blah, blah,' and 'It's got all this extra cushioning and protection.' But then all of a sudden minimalism is the way to go. When you've been around awhile, you just kind of hold your head and go, 'Oh my gosh.' "

As Kayser's collection shows, many minimalist shoe features marketed today as innovations were present decades ago. The outsole of the Tiger Obori, which came out in the early 1970s, wrapped around the upper in the outside ball of the foot area. The outsole also, bizarrely, extended a third of the way up the heel counter. More significantly, the heel was slightly undercut—the heel counter extended slightly over the back of the outsole. Today some minimalist shoes have this design to move runners away from a heavy heel landing.

The Lydiard Road Runner that we met at the beginning of this chapter had an asymmetrical, wide forefoot. Then, as now, this design was touted as allowing more natural foot motion by letting the toes spread and push off optimally. Etonic and Nike models from the 1970s had side lacing, to take pressure off the top of the foot. In the late 1960s, a British shoe was advertised with the tagline "run barefoot on the road." And almost 60 years before *Born to Run* and Vibram FiveFingers became bestsellers, a Japanese runner named Shigeki Tanaka won the 1951 Boston Marathon in shoes that had a separate compartment for his big toe. "I don't want to sound cynical," Kayser says, "but it's all been done."

I asked Kayser if he's ever tempted to run in shoes from his collection. "No," he said, "it's hard to put most of them on. Over time they get stiff. Some of them might fall apart. Some of the ones on my shoe tree started delaminating. The soles and uppers were coming off."

He has another reason not to run in the shoes of his salad days. "My knees hurt so much," Kayser says. "Back then you didn't realize how much pounding your body took in those shoes because you were young and springy. I thought I was indestructible." Kayser and his friend Phil Stewart, race director of the Cherry Blossom 10-miler in Washington, DC, and a 2:19 marathoner in the 1970s, often discuss minimalism. Stewart, in his 60s and still a daily runner, tells Kayser, "I need cushioning!"

WHEN BIGGER WAS BETTER

That desire for cushioning existed in the '70s. The Nike LD 1000, for example, came out in 1976 and had a high, flared heel and plush midsole. "I remember the first time I tried them on," Kayser says. I thought, 'Oh my god, this is wonderful.' When running started getting more popular and the more cushioned shoes started coming out, that was a godsend."

The first running boom, underscored by Jim Fixx's *Complete Book of Running* hitting number one on bestseller lists, broadened the sport's demographics. The average *Runner's World* subscriber who submitted comments in 1971 for *All About Distance Running Shoes* was a 29-year-old male who weighed 145 pounds. Within the decade, the running population started looking much more like the American population.

Longtime runners like Kayser and Stewart appreciated shoes like the LD 1000 because they were such a contrast to the thin models

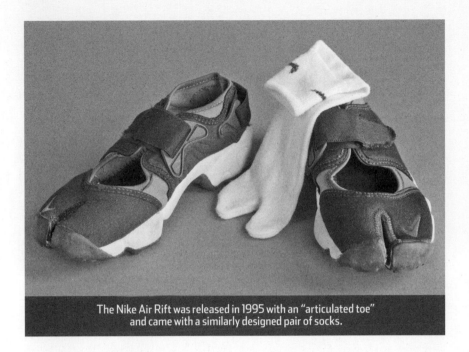

The Nike Air Rift was released in 1995 with an "articulated toe" and came with a similarly designed pair of socks.

they'd been pounding the pavement with for years. New runners—and increasingly, nonrunners—responded to the more cushioned shoes' immediate running-on-pillows sensation when they tried them on. An arms race in cushioning developed among companies hoping to capture that market.

Bob Roncker has been a runner since 1958 and owns four running stores in the Cincinnati area. His running shoe collection trumps even Kayser's; most of the 300 models in it are on display at one of his stores. "When you look at the evolution of shoes in our museum," he says, "you see no flare, then a little flare, then all of a sudden a lot of flare after the Nike LD 1000."

Shoe companies were motivated by more than customer try-on satisfaction. "The thought was that higher heel heights would decrease Achilles tendinitis," says Joe Rubio, a partner in the online running store RunningWarehouse.com. Despite the lack of scientific evidence in support, cushioned soles were said to reduce common running injuries stemming from repetitive impact forces.

Thickly cushioned shoes were also touted as preventing foot-strike hemolysis, or the breakdown of red blood cells in the feet. "That was a large impetus for more cushioned shoes and greater amounts of padding—preventing elite athletes from getting ane-mic," says Rubio. That benefit hasn't been proven. Knowledgeable minimalists such as college biology professor Peter Larson say that the shift in footstrike most minimalists achieve should eliminate concern about footstrike hemolysis. "Impact would seem to be the

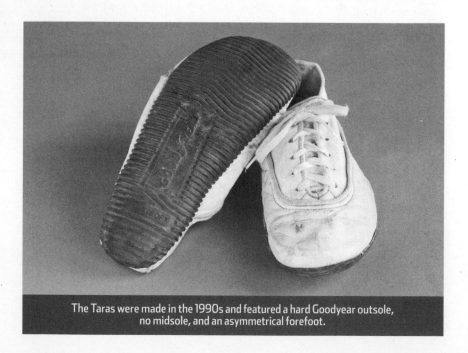

The Taras were made in the 1990s and featured a hard Goodyear outsole, no midsole, and an asymmetrical forefoot.

major driver of hemolysis, and this is vastly reduced among forefoot-strikers relative to heel-strikers."

Even though shoes kept getting bigger in the 1980s and '90s, companies occasionally released models that today's minimalists might smile upon. In 1995, Nike put out the Air Rift. Its distinguishing feature was what Nike called an "articulated toe," by which they meant a separate compartment for the big toe, like the shoes Shigeki Tanaka wore to win the 1951 Boston Marathon. In this case, Nike said the design was inspired by Kenyan runners who grew up barefoot; the shoe, Nike said, helped you run with more of a barefoot gait. The shoes were secured across the top of the foot and behind the heel with Velcro straps, and much of the upper was open. They came with a pair of socks with a separate compartment for the big toe.

The Air Rift was, I thought, a delight to run in and, as so often happens with such shoes, was soon taken off the market. Nike never got around to explaining why, if the articulated-toe design improved performance, it wasn't made standard throughout its running line, or even maintained in one shoe.

A year before the Air Rift came out, the owner of a California running store called Movin' Shoes sent me a pair of oddities called the Taras. (Yes, they were named after the Tarahumara. See "The Tarahumara through the Years" on page 48.) The shoes have a leather upper, a thin, ridged outsole of Goodyear rubber, and a wide, asymmetrical forefoot to match the natural shape of the foot. There's no real heel or forefoot height to measure. One of my size-9.5 models weighs a bit more than 5 ounces. At the time, they retailed for $85.

After I did some running in the Taras, I called the owner to let him know how much I liked them, especially the generous forefoot,

THE TARAHUMARA THROUGH THE YEARS

For a lost tribe, the Tarahumara sure do get written about a lot.

The Mexican tribe of runners central to Christopher McDougall's 2009 book *Born to Run* have been part of running lore for decades. Running historian Roger Robinson notes that former British elite runner Bruce Tulloh visited the Tarahumara in 1971 and wrote articles about them for a British newspaper. Another elite Brit, Tim Johnston, lived in Mexico in 1967 to train for the 1968 Olympic Marathon, held in Mexico City. He told Robinson about his interactions with the Tarahumara: "They were with the Mexican pre-Olympic squad, happy to have nothing to do but run all day, but they were very slow, just shuffling along in traditional huaraches."

A 1976 book, *The Joy of Running*, by Thaddeus Kostrubala, MD, includes sections on the Tarahumara, as well as speculation about running's role in human evolution. The following year, the March 1977 issue of *Running Times* included an interview with Jonathon Cassel, who, the magazine noted, "spent several months living with the Tarahumara." Cassel related stories of—see if this sounds familiar— persistence hunting and running as transportation. "Wherever they go, whether it is across the canyon or 100 yards or 200 miles, they run," Cassel said. "They chase down the game for food, they run wherever they go, their only sport or entertainment is a race in which, of course, they run— and this could be upward of 175 miles."

When I started reading running magazines in the early 1980s, the Tarahumara were presented more as common knowledge than as a paradigm-changing discovery. In 1993 and 1994, many runners now know, members of the Tarahumara won the Leadville Trail 100 Run, a 100-miler in Colorado. Many runners also know that aptitude in trail ultras at altitude is one of several forms of running competency, not the *ne plus ultra* of athletic accomplishment.

As Robinson puts it, "We have long been familiar with the Tarahumara Indians . . . their prowess and their limitations as runners are well known in the running world."

given how wide my feet are. He said the shoes were selling well. Satisfied customers would often report, "The shoes work great!" to which he would respond, "It's not the shoes, it's your feet!"

BAREFOOT RUNNING: LONG COMMON

Ah yes, the feet.

It shouldn't be surprising to find college runners doing barefoot strides even if their team is sponsored by Nike. Rather than a mild form of protest against the shoes, that's simply what competitive runners have done for decades.

The most famous barefoot running accomplishment, of course, is Ethiopian Abebe Bikila's victory at the 1960 Olympic Marathon in Rome. People trying to temper the enthusiasm of barefoot runners often point out that when Bikila repeated as Olympic Marathon champion 4 years later, he wore shoes, and ran faster, as if that one data point has a canceling effect on his barefoot win in 1960. A better view is that, like any intelligent competitive runner, Bikila did what he thought gave him the greatest chance of success on the day. He probably would have won shod in 1960 and barefoot in 1964.

Zola Budd of South Africa is the other most famous barefoot elite runner. She won the 1985 and 1986 World Cross-Country Championships barefoot, and wasn't wearing shoes when she and Mary (Decker) Slaney famously tangled in the 1984 Olympic 3000-meter final. (Budd got blamed for many things in this incident, but at least no one could accuse her of spiking her rivals.) Now in her mid-40s and a resident of South Carolina with the last name Pieterse, she's been a spokesperson for Newton running shoes.

All About Distance Running Shoes notes that many British elites of that era often raced barefoot on the track. (Bear in mind that tracks then were almost always made of cinders, not today's more forgiving surfaces.) Among the occasionally barefoot Brits were Ron Hill, who won the Commonwealth, European, and Boston Marathons and set world records for 10 miles, 15 miles, and 25 kilometers; Bruce Tulloh, who set European records at 3 miles and 6 miles; and Jim Hogan, another winner of the European Marathon Championships and a world record holder at 30 kilometers.

It wasn't just elites who regularly ran barefoot, nor was racing the only time runners went unshod. In *All About Distance Running Shoes,* former *Runner's World* editor Joe Henderson reflected on his high school running in the late 1950s in Iowa, where he was a state champion.

"In that era, running shoes were poorly constructed, cumbersome, and expensive," Henderson wrote a decade after graduating from high school. "I naturally chose not to wear any shoes when running if I could help it. No one on our cross-country team wore them. We trained on the dirt and grass. Our feet got as tough as the soles of some of the shoes I now pay $20 for."

In the 1971 booklet, Henderson lamented that high schools had recently made it mandatory to wear shoes while competing. "International rules have no such requirement," he pointed out wistfully.

As the shoes of the time improved and most adult runners participated in road racing—not track and cross-country—regular barefoot running declined. This didn't make Henderson happy. "We've become so civilized in the 1970s that the sight of a barefoot runner is considered foolhardy, odd, abnormal," he wrote. "This is particularly true if he's seen racing on the roads."

The *All About Distance Running Shoes* survey asked respondents if they ever ran barefoot. "Probably 99.9 percent said no," Henderson wrote. But as one respondent, Dick Cordone, put it, "If the prices of shoes keep going up, I might be forced to."

CHAPTER **4**

FACTS ON FORM, FOOTSTRIKE, AND FOOTWEAR

What research shows—and doesn't show—
about running shoes, injury rates,
barefoot running, and more

"NOBODY KNOWS ANYTHING," screenwriter William Goldman is said to have quipped about Hollywood. If Goldman had been commenting on running-shoe research, he might instead have said, "Nobody can prove anything."

People trying to convince others of minimalism's benefits or risks often cite research to back their claims. This study proves barefoot running is best, that study proves running shoes with heels cause injuries, and so on. Unfortunately, the presentation of the research is often lacking—findings are misrepresented, taken out of context, or given conclusions that aren't in the research. Sometimes all three happen.

This occurs more because people are passionate about the topic and misunderstand the nature of research than because they're being intentionally misleading. But it still doesn't help runners make good decisions.

Here are a few reasons why research on running shoes should be taken in stride:

- The studies are almost always short-term, whereas running is a lifetime sport. Even if you show that something changes over a 10-week study period, that doesn't tell you what continuing that practice for years will do.

- The pool of subjects is often small and of different demographics (age, gender, running history, weekly mileage, etc.) than a lot of runners.

- Study results usually compare mean values between groups. As an individual runner, you may be in line with these mean values, or far afield, and you probably have no way of knowing which is true. As sport podiatrist Kevin Kirby says, "There are many ways to run comfortably and without injury."

- The study design is seldom blind, much less the scientific gold standard of being double-blind (where neither the researchers nor subjects know who's in the experimental group and who's in the control group). If you're running barefoot, you know it. Even acknowledging that the research will have to rely on prospective studies—which follow groups of similar people with one important difference between the groups— it's hard to see how a valid long-term study could be designed. How would you isolate one running-related variable in just one person, not to mention a statistically significant group, over months or years?

- The studies are seldom replicated by other researchers. A key element of scientific research is that others can and do try to replicate your results. This seldom happens with running research, mostly because there's no incentive. As much as we love running, we must admit that whether heeled shoes cause iliotibial band syndrome isn't a top public health priority compared with looking into causes of heart disease.

- Related to the above, the studies are sometimes done or funded by people or companies with a stake in the outcomes. For example, Casey Kerrigan, MD, whose work we'll read about below, has helped a company called OESH design zero-drop shoes. Some of "barefoot professor" Daniel Lieberman's research at Harvard has been funded by Vibram. This isn't as nefarious as it might sound. Potential conflicts of interest are disclosed in peer-reviewed research, and scientists such as Kerrigan and Lieberman don't fudge data. Industry funding isn't inherently bad and can lead to discoveries that might otherwise not be made. But it's undeniable that, for example, Kerrigan has an interest in presenting data that might make you question the merit of conventional running shoes. Researchers who are completely removed from the matter don't have much of an incentive to try to replicate this research.

And from the everyday runner's perspective, here's the most compelling reason to keep all this in perspective: research that shows something doesn't necessarily prove anything.

On that last point, consider one of any number of studies I could cite. A few years ago Kerrigan conducted a study in which she measured external joint torques at the ankle, knee, and hip of people running barefoot and in conventional stability running shoes. When they ran in shoes, the subjects had increased joint torques at the three sites compared with when they ran barefoot.

Greater external joint torques sound bad. It seems reasonable to think that they should lead to greater frequency of injury. But it also sounds reasonable to think that running on soft surfaces is always "safer" than running on hard surfaces, when that's not necessarily so. (More on that below.) Researchers are almost always reluctant—sometimes maddeningly so—to draw big-picture conclusions from their work. Kerrigan hasn't said her finding of greater torque in running shoes proves that conventionally shod runners get injured more often. But the rest of the world isn't that careful, and the researchers aren't in the business of sending out perspective-providing press releases when their work is simplified or taken out of context. So in the case of Kerrigan's torque study, headlines such as "Running Shoes Worse than High Heels" are what people remember. To take another example, a study that Lieberman helped conduct found that heel-strikers on Harvard's cross-country team got injured more than their forefoot-striking teammates. It gets presented by the minimalist shoe company Vivobarefoot's Web site as "It's official—barefoot is best."

None of this helps the average runner make sense of these matters. We hear about these studies most often from nonscientists who cherry-pick research to support a conclusion they've already reached. The more ardent online barefoot advocates don't mention studies like the one published in the *British Journal of Sports Medicine* in 2009 that showed that runners prescribed custom orthotics had less plantar pain over an 8-week period than a control group not running in orthotics. "Ah, but that was a short-term study," the response might be, and that's a valid point. But intellectual honesty compels reading peer-reviewed research consistently. You don't get to tout the results of studies you like but then switch to a design critique of ones you don't like.

Elite coach Steve Magness, who has a master's degree in exercise science and spends his noncoaching hours immersed in this sort of stuff, says, "The research, honestly, hasn't been done to the degree it needs to be done. There's some decent comparative data but there's nothing long-term related to performance or injury prevention that says, 'Here's what minimalism does compared to regular shoes.'"

Any honest assessment of research done to date has to include these three statements:

• Nobody has proven running shoes cause or prevent injuries.

• Nobody has proven running barefoot causes or prevents injuries.

- Nobody has proven that runners who wear conventional running shoes get injured more than barefoot runners or that barefoot runners get injured more than conventionally shod runners.

That doesn't mean the research is worthless (or uninteresting). It's better to be well informed than poorly informed, both in terms of facts and in how to put those facts in context. Below I've summarized some key findings in five topic areas. For a collection of links to the original research, go to www.runnersworld.com/minimalismlinks.

RUNNING SURFACES

Research on running surfaces might not seem the most obvious place to start, but I'm leading with it because the research results lead to another matter of perspective to keep in mind. (As if everything I've laid out so far isn't enough.)

Research consistently shows that runners run differently on different surfaces. Using sensory feedback, we try to regulate impact forces by adjusting footstrike, joint stiffness, and muscle activation based on the firmness of the surface. (Muscle activation refers to the degree of tenseness in muscles before landing.) On harder surfaces such as asphalt, we land more softly than on softer surfaces such as grass.

The most interesting study in this regard involved jumping, not running. People jumped off a bench onto mats of different colors; the colors, they were told, corresponded to different cushioning levels in the mats. When they thought they were jumping on a well-cushioned mat, impact forces were higher than when they thought they were jumping on a less-cushioned mat. This is consistent with the research on adjustments to varying running surfaces. Well, except for one detail: The athletes were lied to—the mats were all equally cushioned. But when they thought they'd be landing on a softer mat, they presumably made subtle adjustments in muscle activation and joint stiffness to let the "softer" mat do some of the work.

This same sort of errant adjustment is thought to occur from wearing cushioned running shoes. Perhaps because of blocked sensory feedback, runners in cushioned shoes stiffen their knees when landing compared to when running barefoot. Impact forces wind up being higher than would be expected; it's as if running in the shoe causes your body to make adjustments that cancel out the supposedly beneficial cushioning.

So the research shows that we make complex, integrated adjustments to account for running surface and what's between us and that surface. Barefoot running on asphalt probably isn't as harsh as it might seem, and running in heavily cushioned shoes on soft surfaces probably isn't as protective as it might seem. Now for the additional bigger-picture thought on research stemming from this.

Nearly all running research of this sort looks at one element in isolation, such as impact forces, joint torque, or running economy. Yet we just saw via one such isolated research focus how the human body while running is an organic whole, with mind and muscles working in sync. This increases the chances of misinterpreting and overemphasizing any one bit of research.

The onus for intellectual honesty in this regard is especially on the most ardent pro-barefoot adherents. They point out, rightfully, that the running body is an amazingly adaptive thing. So why can't those adaptations be made in a healthy way when running in cushioned shoes? Sport podiatrist Stephen Pribut says, "Why do we assume the body suddenly becomes 'dumb' when you put on shoes? Shouldn't we assume it stays smart and makes the correct adjustments?"

MECHANICS OF BAREFOOT AND SHOD RUNNING

The findings on how biomechanics change when running barefoot versus shod are consistent. The best research, such as Lieberman's, includes people who are experienced at running barefoot, rather than just having subjects who always wear shoes suddenly run barefoot. The findings are usually presented as how runners adjust their form when switching from shoes to barefoot, although if you wanted to be persnickety, you could argue it should be the other way around, given that barefoot is the natural state.

When runners ditch their shoes, stride length decreases (by about 6 percent), stride rate increases, and ground-contact time decreases. In Lieberman's famous study published in 2010, runners who were accustomed to conventional running shoes ("the habitually shod," Lieberman called them) were overwhelmingly heel-strikers in their running shoes. When they ran barefoot, they still mostly landed on their heels, but did so with a flatter foot than in their shoes—the angle of dorsiflexion (toes pointed toward the shin) of their feet went from 28 degrees to 16 degrees, and at the ankle went from 9 degrees to a bit over 0 degrees. That last bit means that their ankles were ever so slightly plantarflexed (pointing away from the shin) when they ran barefoot. Meanwhile, the angle at their knee upon landing went from 9 to 12 degrees.

That study also looked at these differences in runners Lieberman called "habitually barefoot"—that is, who regularly ran barefoot or in barefoot-style shoes like the Vibram FiveFingers. (Vibram helped to fund this study.) When running in shoes, half of them landed on their heels, the rest midfoot or forefoot. When barefoot, three-quarters of them used what Lieberman classified as a forefoot strike, and the remaining 25 percent landed on their heels. The joint angles were also quite different from those of the habitually shod. The only situation resulting in dorsiflexion was foot angle when running in shoes, and that was an angle of only 2.2 degrees. Compare that with the 28 degrees of dorsiflexion the habitually shod had in their feet when landing wearing running shoes. The angle of their knee at landing was much more similar barefoot versus shod than was the case with the runners used to conventional running shoes.

This is perhaps the most interesting finding of the study, suggesting that regular barefoot or minimalist runners have what are thought to be better foot and ankle mechanics regardless of what they wear on any one run. We'll return to this notion in Chapter 8.

It's worth remembering that this study, published in *Nature* and given huge amounts of mainstream press, had a small subject pool. There were eight runners in each of the habitually shod and habitually barefoot groups. So when you say half of the habitually barefoot were heel-strikers in shoes but only 25 percent were when barefoot, bear in mind you're talking about changes in two runners.

RUNNING ECONOMY

Things seem pretty straightforward concerning how shoes affect running economy, or the oxygen "cost" of running a given pace.

One commonly cited finding is that every 100 grams (just more than 3.5 ounces) of weight added to a bare foot increases the oxygen cost of running 7:00 mile pace by 1.2 percent. Another is that shoes constituting 1 percent of a runner's weight increase oxygen cost by 3.1 percent. (That would mean 12-ounce trainers for a 150-pound runner.) Another fun one to throw around is that models weighing just over 12 ounces per shoe increase the oxygen cost of running 8:00 mile pace by 4.7 percent. A recent study from Lieberman's lab looked not at bare feet versus shoes, but at FiveFingers versus the Asics Cumulus (a typical conventional running shoe). Regardless of whether they were forefoot- or rearfoot-striking, the runners were 2 to 3 percent more economical in the FiveFingers.

Competitive runners have known this intuitively for years. It's why someone sponsored by Asics might train in the Cumulus (11.2 ounces in a men's size 9), wear the Hyperspeed (7 ounces) for a marathon, and switch to the Piranha (4.7 ounces) for a 5-K.

As for why more runners without shoe contracts don't race barefoot, note that research on running economy hasn't been conducted with large numbers of runners moving at race pace. It's possible the shorter stride most runners adopt barefoot limits performance once you're going faster than a certain race pace. We'll consider this idea more in Chapter 7.

Also, recent research has suggested there's not necessarily a predictable decrease in economy as you move from barefoot to light shoe to heavy shoe. A study from the University of Colorado published in 2012 measured running economy in a small (12) group of men who were midfoot-strikers and used to running barefoot. The researchers measured running economy when the runners ran 8:00 mile pace "barefoot" (actually, they wore thin yoga socks) and in the Nike Mayfly, a racing shoe that weighs a bit more than 5 ounces. Eight of the runners were more economical in the Mayfly, four weren't, and when the results were pooled (as they always are), the difference in running economy when they were "barefoot" compared to in the Mayflys wasn't statistically significant.

By now you're probably tired of my offering five caveats for every research result. So I'll just say that while the Colorado study is interesting and intriguing, it's another example of a small study with precise parameters that gets spun into a supposed game-changer. For example, I'm chagrined to report that the *Running Times* Web site linked to the study with the headline "Here's Proof Barefoot Isn't Better."

INJURY CAUSES AND RATES

This is where things start to get really hazy.

To date, there have been no studies with satisfyingly clear conclusions on why runners get hurt. One research review—meaning that the study authors surveyed existing research to find commonalities—resulted in "strong evidence" for two culprits in lower-leg injuries: mileage and a history of injury. So, one of the leading contributors to injury is having been injured; that clarifies that!

The impact forces of running would seem to be a likely explanation for injury. Except that they're not. Some studies have suggested that runners with what the researchers call "higher vertical loading rate" have more of some injuries, including stress fractures. But other studies have found fewer injuries in runners with a higher vertical loading rate than in those with lower impact forces. As Kirby points out, research has also found seemingly counterintuitive results—such as that running on hard surfaces doesn't lead to more injuries than running on soft surfaces (see the earlier section "Running Surfaces") and that cushioned insoles don't appear to reduce the incidence of stress fractures. Further muddying things is that isolating a primary cause of one type of injury wouldn't necessarily say anything about other injuries. Stress fractures likely have different causes than the rusty-coil sensation many longtime runners feel at their hamstring insertions.

The study on Harvard cross-country runners—the one that Vivobarefoot says makes it official that "barefoot is best"—looked at form, not forces, for insight on injuries. Of the 52 runners in the study, 36 were said to be primarily heel-strikers, the others forefoot-strikers. Nearly three-quarters of the team members were said to get injured every year, and the rearfoot-strikers had roughly twice as many repetitive stress injuries as the forefoot-strikers.

This sounds pretty clear-cut. (Vivobarefoot certainly thinks so.) But as usual, this really just leads to more questions. Maybe the heel-strikers are injured more often because they have some structural weakness that leads them to heel-strike and that would be present no matter how they run. Maybe heel-striking isn't as good as forefoot-striking when you're training for and racing in collegiate cross-country races, but is if your focus in running is elsewhere. Who knows, maybe if the Harvard cross-country team switched to road ultras, the forefoot-strikers would be the ones getting injured more often. And maybe we shouldn't draw grand conclusions from a study on 52 thin runners in their early 20s.

Even if we could prove what causes injury, there's another reason to be leery of leaning too heavily on research on the topic.

A common element of the most rigorous scientific paper and the most superficial newspaper article on minimalism is some version of the statement "Every year, between X and Y percent of runners get injured." The numbers used for X and Y vary significantly, from less than 20 percent at the low end to more than 80 percent at the high end. The numbers are unsatisfactorily vague for a good reason: Nobody can say with confidence how many runners get injured every year.

There are several reasons why. First, there's no commonly agreed-upon definition of an injury. Does it mean an overuse injury bad enough to merit time off from running? That's a reasonable definition, but is it explained as such when runners are asked how often they're injured?

Second, even if that were the universal definition, it's flawed as a means of gathering meaningful data. What might lead you to take a week off from running could be the sort of condition I try to run through. Pushed to its extreme, the definition would mean that people who have running streaks never get injured, because they

MEET A MINIMALIST

PAUL MANGO
SEATTLE, WASHINGTON

Paul Mango's story is a good example of how minimalism can help with, but not necessarily solve, long-simmering injury issues.

Mango began running in ninth grade in the early 1990s, competed throughout high school and part of college, and has been a runner ever since. While training 25 to 35 miles a week and recording PRs such as 18:49 for 5-K and 30:55 for 8-K, he encountered typical bodily complaints; iliotibial band issues have been his greatest challenge.

While running in conventional shoes, Mango always had knee pain when he ran more than 12 miles. Figuring more support and cushioning would help, he moved from

conventional but not massive Asics 2100-series shoes to the Asics Nimbus, then on up to the even heftier Asics Kayano. His knee pain didn't go away, and his iliotibial band started to bother him. He began to see a physical therapist.

While waiting in the therapist's office one day in the fall of 2010, he read an article about Vibram FiveFingers. Soon after, he read an Internet debate on barefoot running. "That's when I decided to give minimalist running a shot," Mango says. "I figured that wearing minimalist shoes would help strengthen my feet and calves, reduce the pain in my knees on long runs, and let me run with better form. I figured that if my lower never miss a day. So, if you don't want to get injured, start a running streak!

Third, this is by necessity self-reported data. Even if there were a universal definition of injury, and even if all runners had the same standard for taking time off because of injury, not all runners have

limbs were stronger and I ran with better form, my IT band issues would go away."

Mango transitioned gradually, starting with one or two runs a week and switching to full-time after a couple of months. His IT band issue subsided.

In the spring of 2011, however, Mango twisted his ankle during a 20-mile trail race. "It was pretty sore after the race, but by the time I got home, I could barely walk back from my car to my apartment. I saw a doctor, and he said that I'd suffered a stress fracture in my foot. One thing I learned from that is that I should've worn a more protective shoe to keep the rocks in the trail at bay and to be more aware of the pain

in my body. Muscle soreness is one thing, but any pain in the joints is a big red flag."

Mango suffered a couple of minor setbacks while returning from the trail-race injury, because of trying to increase mileage and intensity too soon. And his IT band still bothers him some.

"One thing that I've learned from switching to minimalist running is that it exposes a lot of your weak points," he says. "I've learned that I need to regularly do cross-training to strengthen my whole body. Having a good core and strengthening the muscles around your legs, especially the hips, can really help a lot in staying injury-free."

accurate records of all their runs. Without a log, can you say how many days you ran in 2010 and how many days you missed to injury?

All of this drifts even farther away from accuracy when people try to compare injury rates over time. As we saw in Chapter 3, the average *Runner's World* subscriber in the early 1970s was a 145-pound 29-year-old man who ran 50 miles per week. The demographics of running have fundamentally changed since then. Today's *Runner's World* subscribers are evenly split between men and women, with an average age of 42 and average weekly mileage of 20. Today there are more older runners, more new runners, more slow runners, and, let's face it, more runners who weigh more than 145 pounds. Even if accurate injury rates for a given year were possible, comparing them from year to year, not to mention decade to decade, would be meaningless.

Do runners get injured? Of course. Do we know why? Not really. Do we know how many runners got injured last year, and how that compares with how many got injured 5, 10, or 30 years ago? No. Take with a healthy dose of salt any advice on how to proceed in running that's based on injury research.

FORCES AT FOOTSTRIKE

And now we enter the black hole of running research.

What impact forces the body incurs, and how those forces are incurred, is where online discussions of minimalism often deteriorate into people shouting past each other. For those who enjoy spending time arguing such things, there's good news: Both sides can cite research to support their claims. Some studies show that vertical loading rates from impact forces are greater when you run in shoes. Other studies show that vertical loading rates from impact forces are greater when you run barefoot.

One part of this topic that's often discussed is differences in what peak impact forces are like in a heel landing versus a midfoot landing. (This often gets interchanged with what happens when running in conventional shoes versus barefoot.) Lieberman's famous study published in *Nature* included data that peak vertical impact forces were about three times less in forefoot-striking runners who were used to running barefoot, compared with heel-striking runners used to running in conventional shoes. Overall, Lieberman wrote, "in the majority of [forefoot-striking] runners, rates of loading were approximately half those of shod [rearfoot-striking] runners."

But, referring to "Injury Causes and Rates" on page 64, these different impact-force measurements might not mean what we tend to think they do. Leading running mechanist Benno Nigg has produced research showing that people with low peak impact forces get injured as often as people with high peak impact forces. (And, of course, we have to consider all the notions about accuracy of reported injury rates. See what I mean about the black hole?) After surveying research on the topic, Nigg wrote, "One cannot conclude that impact forces are important factors in the development of chronic and/or acute running-related injuries." Instead, Nigg proposed, impact forces are "input signals that produce muscle tuning shortly before the next contact with the ground to minimize soft-tissue vibration and/or reduce joint and tendon loading."

One graphic you'll see often if you delve into this topic compares the peak loading rate of a heel strike versus a midfoot strike. The heel-strike visual has a distinct spike upon initial contact, while the midfoot-strike visual shows a much more even distribution of force from landing to toe-off. It's natural to look at the heel-strike visual and envision the heel crashing into the ground and imagine the bad things this causes compared with the visually pleasing midfoot-strike curve.

By now you won't be surprised to hear it's not that simple—some think more impact forces can lead to increased bone density. "What is the proven danger of the initial 'spike' in the rearfoot strike?" Pribut asks. "I've thought this is a 'signal' to the osteo-cytes [a type of cell found in bone] and bone in general to produce more bone."

In the "Running Surfaces" section (see page 58), we saw how the body makes complex, near-instant changes when it's running. Research can offer valuable and interesting insights into isolated aspects of what happens when we run; it's unclear that it'll do more than that any time soon. Certainly runners shouldn't feel compelled to change things because this or that study "proved" something. I'm not big on clichés, and I wish our society as a whole had more respect for science. But what shoes to run in is definitely an area where the "we're all an experiment of one" bromide trumps the latest from the labs.

CHAPTER **5**

THE MANY MODES
OF MINIMALISM

The characteristics and categories
of minimalist shoes

WHAT DO WE MEAN when we talk about minimalist shoes?

As minimalist and barefoot running have exploded in popularity the last few years, most manufacturers have introduced models said to be in that category. But one manufacturer's minimalist model is another manufacturer's idea of a conventional running shoe. And, of course, different runners have different ideas about what minimalism means. Barefoot devotees apply the term only to barely there models such as the Vibram FiveFingers or Merrell Trail Glove, while runners who are used to 14-ounce trainers with high heels call the Saucony Kinvara a minimalist shoe.

Who's right? They all are. Remember, minimalism and barefooting are a means to the end of better running form. If you find that a given shoe within the broad brush of minimalism helps you to achieve that goal, then that's a minimalist shoe for you. Rigid classifications and debates about what is and isn't a minimalist shoe miss the point of why runners should pay attention to the matter in the first place.

That said, there are certain characteristics that most minimalist shoes share. In this chapter, we'll look at those characteristics and how they can be combined to produce a few broad categories under the minimalism umbrella. In doing so, we'll see how minimalism applies to trail shoes. We'll also examine a question many longtime runners have: If you want to run in a light, low-to-the-ground shoe that encourages getting off your heels, why not just do all your training in racing flats?

THE MARKS OF A MINIMALIST SHOE

Ask 100 people to define the phrase "serious runner," and you'll get at least 30 different answers. Some will emphasize speed, others distance. Some will focus on competitive record, others daily dedication. But when considering any one runner, most people would get to their answer not through some theoretical definition, but by the way Supreme Court Justice Potter Stewart defined pornography—you know it when you see it.

That thinking is applicable to minimalist shoes—you know one when you see it. So in the following description of shared characteristics among minimalist shoes, I'm working more from the standpoint of "What do shoes most people consider minimalist have in common?" than "For a shoe to be considered minimalist, it must meet these criteria or we're not going to talk about it." The former approach not only broadens the types of shoes to consider, but also gets us past arguments about shoe specifics so that we can concentrate on the more important matter of which shoe is right for you.

Here are the key characteristics that most minimalist running shoes have to some degree. Some characteristics will be more important to some runners than others. And some shoes will have more of some characteristics and less of others. That's good, because it increases the chances of finding one that's right for where you are in your minimalist adventure.

Low to the ground. Minimalist shoes have less foam or other material between you and the ground than do conventional running shoes. What's known as a lower "stack height" results in better road feel and encourages your feet to work more naturally. A higher stack height potentially introduces instability, because there's that much more between your proprioceptive muscles and the ground. Look for heels that are less than around 25 millimeters high and a forefoot height not greater than around 17 millimeters, while bearing in mind these are general guidelines rather than deal-breakers for a given shoe.

Not much difference between heel and forefoot height. The difference between a shoe's heel height and forefoot height is known as the ramp angle. Research has shown that too great a ramp angle—as found in most conventional running shoes—can lead to overstriding, heel landing in runners who might otherwise be midfoot-strikers, and other undesirable aspects of running form.

Most minimalist models retain a slightly higher heel than forefoot. Even more moderate "transitional" shoes—conventional-looking models that many runners use to experiment with minimalism—can have just a slight ramp angle. The Saucony Kinvara, for example, has a reported 4-millimeter drop from heel to forefoot, while the Brooks PureConnect has a reported 5-millimeter drop. (Note that these are the measurements reported by manufacturers. Measurements in the *Runner's World* Shoe Lab often yield different values, such as a 7-millimeter drop for the Kinvara and a 4-millimeter drop for the PureConnect.)

A few shoes, such as most Altras and Merrells, are what are known as "zero-drop," meaning no difference between heel and forefoot height.

Light weight. As noted in Chapter 4, too much weight on your feet reduces your running economy. Almost by definition, minimalist shoes should be among the lightest models on the market. As a general guideline, think less than 9 ounces for a men's size 9 and less than 8 ounces for a women's size 8.

A simple upper. The top part of your shoe should do little more than secure your foot to the bottom of the shoe. Thick overlays and heavily padded tongues add weight without increasing performance.

A wider-than-average toebox. Many conventional running shoes (as well as many racing flats) taper at the front of the shoe.

BRANDON WOOD
ANCHORAGE, ALASKA

Brandon Wood became a minimalist not long after he became a runner. Initial overeagerness toward running in general and switching to less shoe left him licking his wounds, but now he's found a middle ground sustainable for the long run.

Wood ran his first marathon in December 2010 at age 28, less than a year after becoming what he considers a regular runner. After that race, he was sidelined for a month and a half with an iliotibial band injury. "During those 6 weeks, I was going crazy and began reading everything I could about injuries, running form, minimalist shoes, etc.," he says. "One thing that kept coming up again and again was the shoes I was wearing, and it got me thinking that switching to a more minimal shoe may be the key."

Unfortunately, Wood's body wasn't prepared to handle his understandable enthusiasm that he'd found a solution. "I bought into the hype, and I dove headfirst into minimal running," he says. "I bought a pair of Vibram FiveFingers and began running in them regularly. I broke the cardinal rule,

doing too much too soon, and almost injured myself again with a metatarsal fracture. After that, I regrouped and reassessed my thinking.

"The second time around, I took a much more sane and gradual approach to transitioning to minimal shoes. Today, I run most of my miles in shoes like the Saucony Kinvara and Altra Instinct—both relatively minimal shoes, but they still offer some cushioning." Wood does about 75 percent of his 30 to 40 weekly miles in those models, and uses a heavier Montrail shoe for trail running.

Wood looks at what he calls "this happy medium" solely as a means to the end of injury-free running. Although he says he likes the feel of minimal shoes, especially the wide toebox of the Altra Instinct, that's still more a functional appreciation than anything else. "My initial motivation was injury prevention, and that's pretty much what continues to drive this decision for me," he says. "If running in minimal shoes hadn't helped me stay injury-free through four marathons, I would be looking at other solutions."

MEET A MINIMALIST

This horribly conceived design inhibits your foot's natural flexion in the forward arch and constrains your toes' ability to splay. When arch flexion and toe splaying are allowed, these parts of the foot can better help in propelling you forward. The widest part of most people's feet is across the heads of the metatarsals (toe bones). A shoe designed to encourage a natural running gait should reflect that.

A lack of gadgetry. Running shoe industry mainstays like dual-density midsoles and plastic devices intended to control pronation are exactly what minimalist runners are trying to run away from. These add-ons not only increase a shoe's weight but can also inhibit the foot's natural motion.

Flexibility. A minimalist shoe ideally should be flexible in two ways—from front to back and from side to side. This allows your foot to move naturally through the gait cycle and to adapt instantly to the different ground conditions you encounter on a typical run.

Information on some of these characteristics is relatively easy to find on your own through manufacturers' Web sites, magazine shoe reviews, and online retailers. (The site RunningWarehouse.com sets the standard for giving stack height and weight for every model it sells.) Other characteristics are harder to judge without seeing and touching the shoe. This can be tricky for many models, as most retailers still lean heavily toward carrying conventional running shoes over a full range of minimalist models.

Also consider that some of the most innovative minimalist shoes, such as Altra, are small companies that have yet to make their way into most stores. In these cases, your best bet is to find a retailer who will work with you on a fair return policy if you decide a shoe won't work for you once you've seen it and tried it on.

MINIMALIST CATEGORIES

Within the broad rubric of minimalism, it's helpful to think of three main categories: barely there/barefoot-style, moderate minimalists, and transitional/gateway shoes. Here's more on each of those categories, again with the caveat that these are general groupings more than distinct silos.

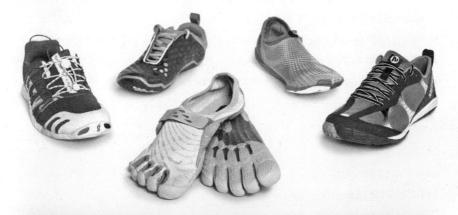

Examples of barefoot-style shoes (clockwise from bottom center): Vibram FiveFingers SeeYa; inov-8 Bare-X Lite 135; Vivobarefoot Evo; Adidas AdiPure Adapt; Merrell Road Glove.

Barely There/Barefoot-Style Shoes

These are the minimalist's minimalists, so to speak. They have the no real midsole to speak of, just an outsole for abrasion resistance, putting your foot no more than 10 millimeters off the ground. They have almost no cushioning. They also have a tiny or nonexistent ramp angle and a wide toebox. The whole idea is to let your foot work as naturally as possible while providing a bit of protection from underfoot items. Examples include the Vibram FiveFingers, Vivobarefoot Evo, and Merrell Road Glove.

Moderate Minimalist Shoes

These shoes share many characteristics of the barely there models, including a slight ramp angle, wide forefoot, and, usually, firm midsole. Their stack height is greater than those of the barefoot-style models but noticeably lower than those of conventional running shoes. Most runners new to minimalism will feel like their mechanics are different in these shoes, but because the shoes

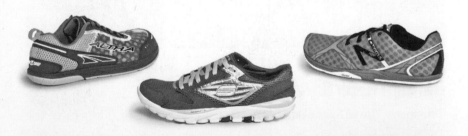

Examples of moderate minimalist shoes (left to right):
Altra Instinct 1.5; Skechers GoRun; New Balance Minimus Road.

retain some elements of conventional running shoes, won't find them to be as abrupt a change as they do the barely there shoes. Examples include the New Balance Minimus Road, Altra Instinct, Nike Free, and Skechers GoRun.

Transitional/Gateway Shoes

These shoes retain many of the features of conventional running shoes, including a relatively high stack height and soft midsole. Their defining feature is a low ramp angle. Many runners use these shoes as their entrée into minimalism—hence the category name— by first adapting to the low ramp angle, then moving closer to the ground in more minimalist models if so inspired. Examples include the Saucony Kinvara, Brooks PureConnect, and Newton Gravitas.

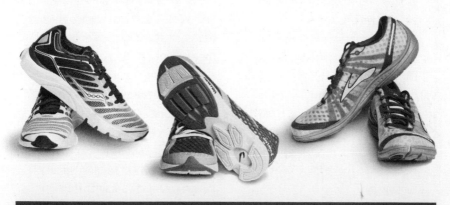

Examples of transitional minimalist shoes (left to right):
Saucony Kinvara; Newton Distance; Brooks PureConnect.

MINIMALISM ON THE TRAIL

In the 1990s, Ann Trason was one of the top ultramarathoners in the world. She won the storied Western States 100-miler 14 times; the course record she set there in 1994 lasted until 2012.

Trason was sponsored by Nike and appeared in an ad for Nike trail shoes in the mid-'90s. So when I spent a few days with her in 1996, I was surprised that for a long run on the Western States trail

ORTHOTICS AND MINIMALISM

Orthotics—customized insoles designed to address an injury or structural weakness—seem antithetical to the let-the-body-do-its-thing ethos of minimalism. Can the two coexist?

Sometimes, says Brian Fullem, DPM, a sport podiatrist in Tampa, Florida, who ran 14:25 for 5-K while competing for Bucknell. If you've been prescribed orthotics, he says, you should consider whether you still need them, regardless of what kind of shoe you're thinking about running in.

"I have a lot of patients come in to see me who say, 'I've been wearing orthotics for 10 years,' and I'll ask them why they got them, and they don't remember," Fullem says. "When I make someone orthotics, it's almost always either to treat a specific injury or because they've had a history of injuries, and I'm trying to correct what I perceive to possibly be the cause of the injury."

If you received orthotics for a given injury but no longer have that injury, Fullem would generally advise weaning yourself off them. If, however, you have an injury in we started together, she had on the Nike Air Skylon T/C, an excellent lightweight road shoe of the time. When I asked her why someone in a Nike trail shoe ad was going to do a 44-mile (!) trail run in road shoes, she said, "A good shoe is a good shoe."

So take it from Trason, not me: A good shoe for running on the roads should also work well on trails. Trason's comment was especially pertinent in the mid-'90s. Companies were just starting to introduce trail running shoes, most of which were more hiking boot

the acute phase, he advises continuing to wear orthotics and holding off on experimenting with minimalism until the injury is resolved.

"I'll give you a specific example— the posterior tibial tendon," he says. "The posterior tibial tendon helps to support the arch. If it's injured, a little tendon like the posterior tibial tendon can't resist the hundreds of pounds of force that happen every time you land running. I'm sorry, but doing drills and strengthening your foot and running in a Vibram FiveFingers isn't going to help you overcome that

injury while it's acute, I believe.

"I think the same is true with something like plantar fasciitis. Let's get rid of the inflammation first. Once the injury is better, then start thinking about switching to a minimalist shoe."

If you have a pattern of injury but aren't currently in an acute phase, Fullem still advises sticking with the orthotics you've been prescribed to deal with that problem. Over time, through strengthening work and reaping some of the benefits of minimalism, you should be able to transition out of the orthotics.

than performance-oriented running shoe. The heavy, sturdy shoes seemed counterintuitive—on trails, wouldn't you want something that much more flexible, nimble, and low to the ground to help quickly adjust to varying terrain?

Since then, trail running shoes have markedly improved, but it really took the minimalist movement to get trail shoes toward what they should have been from the start. Now you can find the same range of minimalist trail shoes—from barely there to borderline conventional—as you can road shoes. Of course, Trason's tenet still holds. But if you are interested in minimalist trail shoes, what should you look for?

TRAIL SHOES VS. ROAD SHOES

The first thing to consider is the difference between a road shoe and a trail shoe. The largest difference is usually in the outsole. A trail shoe is going to have a more rugged, aggressive design to better handle the constantly changing surface underfoot.

Before minimalist trail shoes were widely available, I tried some trail runs in road racing flats, on the theory that their light, flexible construction would give me greater agility over roots and rocks. And they did. But the flat, uncontoured outsole of the racing shoes also meant that I felt every root and rock I stepped on. These weren't the most enjoyable trail runs of my life—if I wasn't landing on something hard and sharp, I was cherry-picking my way down the trail in more of a prancing than running motion. Some trail shoes have a rock plate, a thin layer of reinforced material directly above the outsole, to allow more cruising and less bruising over tricky terrain.

For similar reasons, trail shoes tend to have more of a protective upper. The reasoning here is that a sturdier wrap across the top of the foot will give greater protection from various rocks and twiggery protruding from the trail and will shelter the side and top of your foot if you roll an ankle while navigating uncertain ground. Reinforced sidewalls are common to help keep trail debris from entering the shoe.

Throw in other features, like a firm midsole to increase stability, and conventional trail running shoes start to outweigh their road-running counterparts by 2 to 3 ounces.

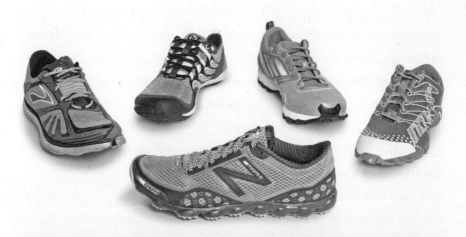

Examples of minimalist trail shoes (clockwise from bottom center): New Balance Minimus Amp; Brooks PureGrit; Merrell Trail Glove; Adidas Adizero XT-10; inov-8 f-lite 230.

MINIMALIST TRAIL SHOES VS. CONVENTIONAL TRAIL SHOES

These days, one of the worst-performing categories in the running-shoe business is traditional trail shoes, while one of the hottest is minimalist trail shoes. One retailer I spoke with lamented that he couldn't unload conventional trail shoes even at liquidation prices.

It makes sense that some of the greatest enthusiasm for minimalism has come from trail runners. What better place to get back to more natural running than in the woods or around a lake or atop a mountain ridge? Also, on a soft surface like a bridle path or the floor of a pine forest, a shoe's lack of cushioning isn't as noticeable as on asphalt. And as I mentioned above, for many runners, traditional trail shoes harmed rather than helped the more agile, no-two-strides-the-same gait that's appropriate on many trails.

That said, I can vouch that less isn't always better on trails. This breakthrough insight stems from some short runs I did in the Maine woods in an early iteration of the Vibram FiveFingers. The experience was much the same as when I ran on the rutted, rooty ground in road flats—at times more of a walk-and-jump motion than something resembling running. Fortunately, there are now plenty of light, flexible, low-to-the-ground shoes with a trail-appropriate outsole.

How minimal to go with a trail shoe depends more on what the trails you run on are like than on the cushioning question that might mostly guide what minimalist road shoe you seek. No matter how adept a trail runner you are, some venues—such as a single-track trail over lots of rocks and roots—are going to get tiresome after a

SOCKS AND MINIMALISM

Whether to wear socks as you experiment with running in less shoe is an individual matter. Going sockless seems to be more in the spirit of letting your feet do their thing free of accretions; some minimalists will tell you that socks, especially thick ones, add another barrier to really feeling and reacting to the ground. A University of Toledo study published in 2011 found that people's single-leg static balance was better barefoot than while wearing thin conventional socks or five-toe socks. Sport podiatrist Brian Fullem, however, says he doesn't think that socks interfere with a runner's proprioception while in motion.

With their elemental design, many minimalist shoes have uppers that shouldn't irritate an otherwise bare foot. Still, even the slightest irritant, like a low toebox rubbing against a nail, can have major consequences by the end of a 2-hour run. Blisters can form when you go sockless, especially when it's hot and your feet are sweating a lot. At other times of the year, going sockless, especially in a highly ventilated shoe, can lead to uncomfortably cold feet, at least at the beginning of your run. (If you doubt me, come on up to Maine for an early-morning run next January.)

Coolmax, merino wool, and other wicking materials in socks help draw sweat away from your feet. "If there is more sweat being absorbed by the shoe, then that might set a person up for a greater chance of getting athlete's foot infections," says Fullem. Odor absorption is another reason to consider socks.

If you're so inspired, experiment with running without socks, but don't feel like you're less of a minimalist if you revert to wearing them.

while in some of the more barely there models. There's a freedom in trail running that can be diminished by having to be aware of every footplant; if you're running amid great scenery, don't you want to be able to look around at times? There are enough minimalist trail models available that you should be able to find a happy medium between a close-to-barefoot feel and enough underfoot protection so that you can lose yourself in the run.

WHAT ABOUT RACING SHOES?

In the early years of this century, I found myself gravitating toward doing almost all my running in racing shoes. This wasn't because I was working from a creedal statement of what shoes are acceptable to run in, and it certainly wasn't because I was cranking out daily tempo runs. It was simply that, as training shoes kept getting bigger and bigger, the only widely available models that still felt like shoes I wanted to run in were racing shoes.

I wasn't alone in this solution. Message boards of the time were full of runners sharing advice (and frustrations) on which racing flats worked best as daily trainers. Given where shoes were heading then—toward ever-thicker stack heights and greater ramp angles—saying, "I do all my running in racing shoes" wasn't as dramatic a pronouncement as it might appear. A lot of racing shoes were also trending up in height and weight. Shoes like the original Saucony Fastwitch and the Fila Racer were more or less what lightweight trainers had been a dozen years before.

Now that there's a wide variety of minimalist shoes designed for daily running, does training in racing shoes still make sense?

Given what most people are looking for in a minimalist shoe, yes.

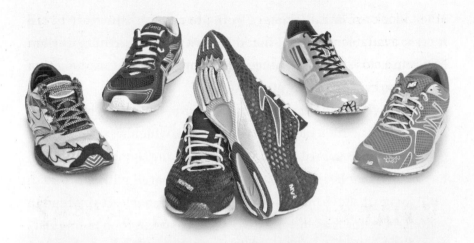

Examples of racing flats (clockwise from bottom center): Newton MV$_2$;
Mizuno Universe; Asics Hyperspeed; Adidas Adizero Hagio; New Balance 1400.

The average racing flat is responsive and low to the ground, and doesn't have much of a ramp angle. Consider something like the Asics Hyperspeed, the shoe that Ryan Hall races marathons in. In a men's size 9, it weighs 7 ounces and has a stack height of 21 millimeters in the heel and 15 millimeters in the forefoot. Now consider the first generation of the New Balance Minimus Road, one of the poster children of mainstream minimalism. In a men's size 9, it weighs 8 ounces and has a stack height of 19 millimeters in the heel and 14 millimeters in the forefoot. The Hyperspeed is marketed as a racing shoe, the Minimus Road as a daily trainer, but in terms of two of the most important factors minimalists look for in a shoe, there's not much to distinguish the two models.

At the really minimal end of the spectrum, to most people a racing flat like the Mizuno Wave Universe (4 ounces in a men's size 9, stack height of 19 millimeters in the heel, 14 millimeters in the forefoot) isn't going to feel that different from something like the Merrell Road Glove (6.9 ounces in a men's size 9, stack height of 11 millimeters in the heel and forefoot).

A few caveats: One way that manufacturers keep weight down in racing flats is with a blown rubber outsole, which wears out more quickly than a standard outsole. Then again, the Hyperspeed, which has a blown rubber outsole, costs $75, compared with more than $100 for most shoes marketed as minimalist models. If you tend to switch shoes for reasons other than outsole wear, then racing flats can make good financial sense as an everyday option.

Perhaps more important for many minimalists' purposes, many racing flats are built on a traditional spike last (basically, the mold or skeleton around which the shoe is built). Models made this way tend to taper toward the front of the foot and have a low toebox. This is in contrast to the wide forefoot that's a key part of the design of many minimalist shoes. (Why racing flats, which are supposedly created to encourage best-possible mechanics, retain a design that inhibits natural foot motion remains a mystery.)

Also, many racing flats have a higher ramp angle than even the gateway minimalist shoes. For example, the Adidas Adios 2, which Patrick Makau wore to set a marathon world record at Berlin in 2011, has a heel-to-toe differential of 9 millimeters, compared with a 4-millimeter drop for the Saucony Kinvara or 5-millimeter drop for the Brooks PureFlow.

Put simply, consider racing shoes as an option when deciding on a minimalist shoe, even if you never intend to compete. As we'll see in the next section, the best approach is to focus on criteria, not category, when deciding what shoes are best for you.

What Shoe Is Right for You?

We've just spent several pages looking at various categories of minimalist shoes. That's good and necessary information, because it's important to know your options and the thinking that goes into them. But as we saw with racing shoes, sometimes shoes are in a given category more because of a company's way of looking at the world than because of where they fit in with everything else on the market. When you go to buy a minimalist shoe, your best bet is to look past rigid categories and focus on which characteristics matter most to you.

A personal example: If I had to pick one running shoe from the last $3\frac{1}{2}$ decades as my favorite, it would be the first generation of the Brooks Cheetah. Marketed as a lightweight trainer, it came out in the early 1990s. It was low to the ground and had a minimal ramp angle, a wide forefoot, and, for me, just the right combination of responsiveness and cushioning. So of course in 1996 Brooks nearly doubled the height of the midsole in the next iteration, the Cheetah 2. It was the same shoe in name only. I bought 10 pairs of the originals and mourned the day I retired the last pair.

Remembering what I loved about the Cheetah helps me pick shoes now. If a shoe's midsole is toward the firm end of things, I know I'll wish for a little more softness. If the ramp angle and stack height are much greater than in the Cheetah, I know I'll feel tilted forward and suspended above the ground. If the weight is much more than that of the Cheetah, I know I won't have that free-floating feeling, especially at the end of long runs or when I'm tired.

It's not that I have Brooks Cheetah stats lying around that I compare all shoes with. Rather, knowing that the Cheetah was, to date, the best shoe for me ever designed, I can quickly assess how closely other shoes come to its combination of attributes. Whether a particular model is marketed as a lightweight trainer or racing flat or minimalist shoe is irrelevant. Rather, based on knowing what's most important to me, I try to find a shoe from what's available that feels like the closest match to my memory of the Cheetah. Sometimes that's what's marketed as a minimalist shoe, sometimes it's what's marketed as a lightweight trainer, and sometimes it's what's marketed as a racing flat.

You should take the same approach when trying to choose from among the broad array of minimalist shoes. Of course, if you've always worn conventional running shoes, there will be some differences as you move toward minimalism. Most likely this will have to do with stack height and ramp angle. Still, try to be able to articulate the key features that the running shoes you've most liked have shared. Think about things like:

- Do I like a firm midsole or a soft midsole?

- Do I like a wide toebox or a narrow toebox?

- Do I like a high toebox or a low toebox?

- Do I like a firm heel counter or a soft heel counter?

In an ideal world, you'd then be able to go to a running store, tell them your general preferences, and ask them to bring out the five minimalist models that best match these criteria. Then you could try on each one, see which feels best, and go from there. If you take it home and can run in it without problems, proceed. If you get hurt or the shoe seems to get in the way of enjoyable running, cut your losses and start over.

In the likely case that that's not possible, make use of fellow runners' experiences via message boards and see what magazine shoe reviews and online running shops say about similar models.

But wait, you might be thinking: How do I know how much or how little of a minimalist shoe to look for? How do I know what minimalist shoe I can safely start running in? And, come to think of it, how should I go about starting to run in whatever minimalist shoe I buy?

Determining how ready your body is to start running in minimalist shoes and how to integrate minimalist shoes into your training program is the subject of the next chapter.

CHAPTER 6

STEPS TO MINIMALISM

How to transition safely to running in less shoe

IN MARCH 2012, a woman runner came to sport podiatrist Brian Fullem's office in Tampa, Florida, with a sore foot. While talking with the woman, Fullem suspected she had a stress fracture. He asked her about her running. She said she had recently started training for a marathon and had switched shoes.

"I asked why she'd switched shoes," Fullem says, "and she said, 'I read *Born to Run* and saw we're not supposed to be running in regular shoes, and the Kenyans run barefoot, and so I figured I'd start running in minimalist shoes.'" She had discarded her conventional training shoes to do all her running in a barefoot-style model. Fullem knew what to tell this patient because she wasn't the first such case he'd seen in recent years.

"I told her that you can't just go from wearing running shoes with a 12-millimeter heel-to-toe drop to a shoe that doesn't have any cushioning, any support," he says. "I told her *Born to Run* isn't coming from any sort of science perspective, but from the perspective of telling a story about the Tarahumara, who run all day in these handmade sandals. I told her that's not her, and that there has to be a transition into minimalist shoes."

Up in Washington, DC, and New York City, physiotherapist Phil Wharton was seeing patients with similar pains—and recent histories. "Because of all the awareness, we've seen people jump in too fast or without a proper progression plan," he says about injured would-be minimalists. "Think about it like this: You get a device like this phone I'm using now. I certainly don't read the manual or the fine print. I don't even look at the quick-start guide. I just get it and start using it, and I don't know what I'm doing.

"And that's kind of what's happening with people in minimalism. They remember parts of *Born to Run*. They don't remember the part where Christopher McDougall says he had a personal trainer and did strengthening. What they remember is 'getting into a minimalist shoe changed my life and stopped all these injuries.' And so they just jump right in.

"The biggest pitfall is that we're a culture that's not designed to look at process," Wharton continues. "When we want to do something, we want to do it 100 percent, starting today."

In this chapter, we'll look at a better way of becoming a minimalist than the all-at-once mode that felled Fullem's and Wharton's patients and thousands of other overeager runners. We'll see how to gradually integrate minimalism into your running to minimize your chance of injury and maximize your chance of long-term success.

ARE YOU READY?

As we've seen in earlier chapters, running in shoes that are lower to the ground, more level, and less cushioned than conventional running shoes places different demands on your body. To quickly recap: Your feet need to be stronger, your plantar fasciae and Achilles tendons need to be longer, your postural muscles need to be functioning well, and so on. Even your neuromuscular system needs to be ready to work differently, as you use more proprioceptive feedback than when running in thickly cushioned shoes that blunt those messages among muscles, nerves, and brain.

So why not just suck it up, start running in minimalist shoes, and allow your body to adapt? Wharton puts it this way: "What I see a lot is people wearing minimalist shoes and running with terrible form. So they go to a form clinic and they fix their form. That's going to last about 2 weeks before it wears off because they can't hold their form if their bodies aren't ready. People have to take a step back and make sure their body is working correctly first.

"We know minimalism is good, but here's the rider to the contract," Wharton continues. "The precursor is you gotta make sure your body is working correctly. Otherwise, you're going to get the injuries we see with minimalism. That's where the real gung-ho folks are going to come up against a brick wall if they're not addressing this."

There's enormous variability among runners in how prepared their bodies are for minimalism. This is true even among runners of the same age, gender, build, and lifetime mileage, among other factors. There are, however, a few common limiting factors in runners successfully transitioning to minimalism.

Below are five tests. Some were developed by Wharton, some by physical therapist Jay Dicharry, formerly the director of the SPEED Performance Clinic at the University of Virginia. Each targets one of the prime bodily needs for long-term, injury-free minimalism. If you can pass all these tests, you should have little to no difficulty in transitioning to minimalism if you follow the guidelines laid out later in this chapter.

If you fail a test, that means you're lacking that key aspect of functional strength or flexibility—that is, strength or flexibility directly related to the demands of what you're trying to do. Your chances of getting injured while running barefoot or in minimalist shoes are greater than if you could pass the test and followed the same transition plan. If you currently fail most of the tests, then your road to healthy minimalism will be even longer.

Failing one or more of the tests, however, doesn't mean you're not made for minimalism. After each test you'll see a simple exercise to improve that area of functioning. In some cases you can make dramatic improvements in as little as a week. Almost everyone can eventually get to where they can pass all the tests.

So, as of today, how ready are you to run in minimalist shoes? Let's find out.

TESTS

TEST #1: ANKLE DORSIFLEXION/POSTERIOR CHAIN RANGE OF MOTION

Why test: If your Achilles tendon lacks sufficient flexibility, you not only limit your ability to push off effectively, but also increase your chance of injuring the tendon or surrounding soft tissue. This test also indicates how well your gastrocnemius (outer calf muscle) and hamstrings work together when your ankle is dorsiflexed (pointed toward your shin) and your upper back is flexed; restriction in the calves and hamstrings when the ankle is dorsiflexed will place additional strain on your Achilles tendon.

How to test: Sit with both legs straight on the floor. Lock the knee of the leg you're going to test; keeping your leg straight fixes the

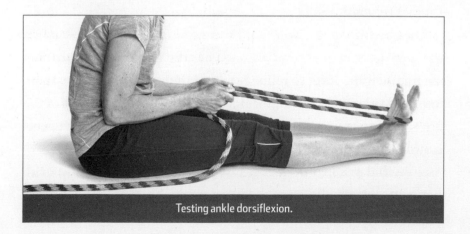

Testing ankle dorsiflexion.

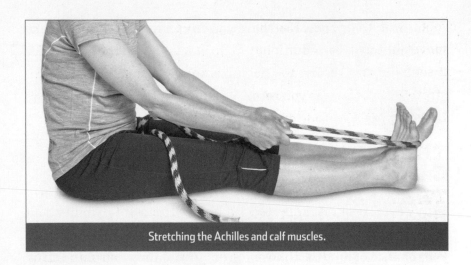

Stretching the Achilles and calf muscles.

hamstring at the knee and pelvis to isolate the gastrocnemius where it inserts at the heel. Loop a strap or towel around the ball of the foot to be tested. Let your thoracic spine (middle to upper back) roll forward naturally and comfortably. Flex your foot toward your shin, using the strap only to gently guide the movement.

To pass this test, your ankle should be able to flex 20 degrees toward your shin, and your upper body should be able to flex 45 degrees forward.

How to improve: Even though the test might seem focused on the Achilles tendon, "what we need here is for the entire gastrocnemius/Achilles lever to relax, reset, and lengthen," says Wharton. Therefore, do the following stretch, which targets both parts of the lever. It's essentially the test exercise, but done gently and repeatedly to gradually lengthen the tissue.

Sit with both legs straight. Loop a strap or towel around the foot of the leg to be stretched and grasp both ends with your hands. Use the muscles in the front of your lower leg to flex your foot toward your knee. Use the strap only to assist at the end of the movement to get an additional slight stretch. Hold the stretch for 2 seconds and return to the starting position. Exhale as you stretch, and inhale as you return the foot to the starting position. Do 10 reps on each side daily.

TEST #2:
BIG-TOE (HALLUX) DORSIFLEXION

Why test: An inability to move your big toe toward your shin can be an indicator of a tight plantar fascia, says Wharton. Poor big-toe dorsiflexion limits your ability to roll through smoothly to toeing off and can make your foot rotate enough to cause lower-leg injuries.

How to test: Sit with your knees bent at 90 degrees and your feet flat on the floor. Slide your hips forward so that your knees are

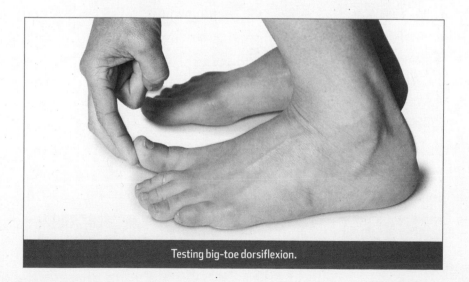

Testing big-toe dorsiflexion.

slightly ahead of your toes. Reach down and grab your big toe while keeping the ball of your foot on the floor.

To pass this test, you should be able to raise your big toe 30 degrees off the floor without the ball of your foot coming off the floor.

How to improve: Use massage rather than stretching to loosen the plantar fascia. Sit with one leg crossed over the other, with the outside ankle of the foot to be massaged on the other knee. Press into the bottom of your foot with your thumbs. Wherever you feel a sore spot, press down for a few seconds while flexing your toes up and down. "The massage needs to be focused pressure where you feel the microbundles of fascia release," says Wharton. Spend a few minutes per foot daily.

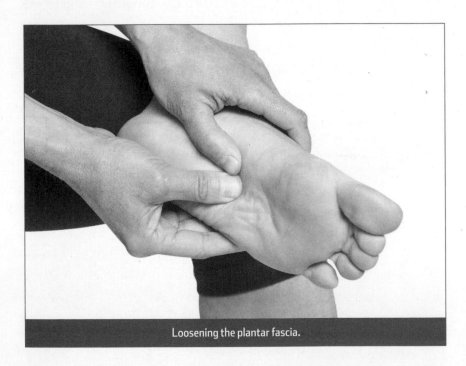

Loosening the plantar fascia.

TEST #3:
BIG-TOE (HALLUX) ISOLATION

Why test: About 85 percent of foot control comes from the big toe, Dicharry says. If your big toe can't operate independently, your foot can't properly adjust itself during the stance phase (between landing and toeing off). An unstable arch will transmit that instability up your leg. "Like the glute is the big push muscle in your hip apparatus, the big toe is the big extensor flexor for your lower leg," Wharton says.

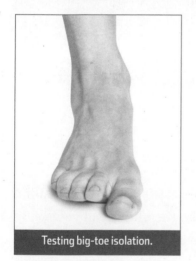

Testing big-toe isolation.

How to test: Stand tall but relaxed. Keep all the toes of one foot on the floor. On the other foot, press the big toe into the floor and raise your other toes while keeping your ankle stable.

To pass this test, you should be able to keep the big toe flat on the ground (instead of bending it) while you raise the other toes, and your ankle shouldn't roll in or out.

How to improve: Increase the flexibility of your toe extensors and flexors. Sit with one leg straight and the other bent at 90 degrees. Grab the toes of the bent leg while keeping the heel on the floor. Curl your toes away from your body, using your hand only to assist gently at the end of the motion. Bring your toes back to the starting position and then curl them toward your body, again using your hand only at the end of the motion. That's 1 repetition. Do 10 repetitions on each foot daily.

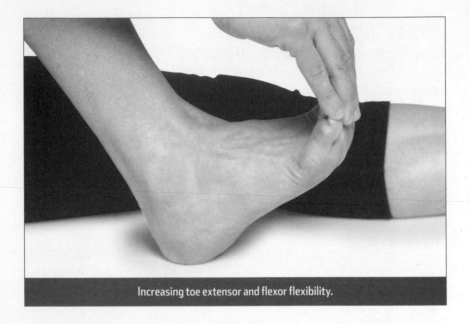
Increasing toe extensor and flexor flexibility.

TEST #4:
ANKLE INVERSION AND EVERSION

Why test: If your ankle can't move adequately toward the midline of your body (inversion) and away from the midline of your body

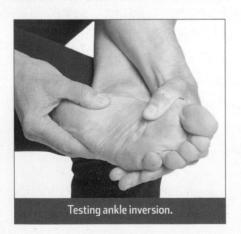
Testing ankle inversion.

(eversion), "you won't utilize your arch's shock absorber or spring to withstand the impact of footstrike," says Wharton.

How to test: Sit with one leg bent at 90 degrees and the outside ankle of the foot to test resting just above the opposite knee. While holding that foot on the outside forefoot, rotate it inward and point the sole of the foot up.

Now bring that foot up so that it's just in front of your butt. From the ankle, rotate the foot outward and away from your body's midline.

To pass the first test, you should be able to rotate your foot inward 15 degrees. To pass the second test, you should be able to rotate your foot outward 5 degrees.

How to improve: Do inversion/eversion walking. First, walk like a pigeon: Turn your feet in toward each other at about 45 degrees while not bending your knees. Taking long strides, walk for 20 yards, staying on the outside of your arches as much as possible. Stop and turn around. Now walk like a duck: Turn your feet away from each other at about 45 degrees while not bending your knees. Taking small strides, walk back the 20 yards to your starting point, staying on the inside of your arches as much as possible. Do two or three of these circuits daily.

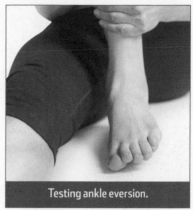

Testing ankle eversion.

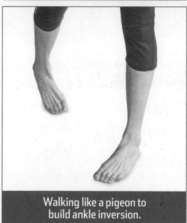

Walking like a pigeon to build ankle inversion.

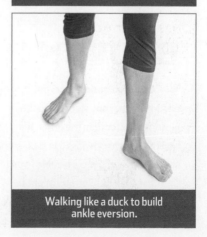

Walking like a duck to build ankle eversion.

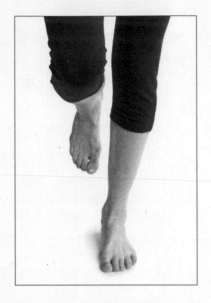

TEST #5:
SINGLE-LEG BALANCE

Why test: Imbalances and weaknesses in your hip and trunk areas introduce instability into your gait and require your feet and lower legs to absorb more impact forces than they should.

How to test: Stand tall but relaxed with your hands on your hips. Lift one leg so that its foot is slightly below the other knee. Keep the heel and the inside and outside of the ball of the foot standing on the floor. Repeat with the other leg.

To pass this test, you should be able to hold the raised-foot position for 30 seconds while keeping your weight evenly distributed over your foot. Your leg and upper body should remain still.

BODY IN BALANCE

While doing these tests, pay attention to whether one side of your body performs better than the other. It's likely that if you can pass a test on one side of your body, you'll be able to on the other side. But you still might be surprised by the differences, which are evidence of imbalances you would do well to address independently of these tests. For example, I do much better on all these tests on my left side. It's no coincidence that almost every lower-leg injury I've had in the last 3½ decades has been in my right leg.

How to improve: Practice the test a few times a day until you can pass it. Once you can hold the position for 30 seconds, try doing it with your eyes closed. You'll be in for a treat!

Let's say you're one of the biomechanically blessed and have passed all the tests. Now you need to decide what shoe to start your transition in, and how to go about safely incorporating it into your running.

How Minimal a Shoe to Start?

As we saw in Chapter 5, the phrase "minimalist shoe" covers a wide range of options among features like heel-to-toe drop, height of midsole, and amount of cushioning. Deciding which minimal shoe to use when starting your transition begins with the general questions noted in Chapter 5, such as whether you like a wide or narrow toebox. Once you've found some options within the broad characteristics you want, then you can decide how minimal a shoe to go to compared with your current one.

There are no hard-and-fast rules here. If you passed the five tests above, you could probably go right to as barefoot-style a shoe as you want, assuming you listen to your body during the transition. If your performance on the tests was shakier, you should probably consider a more gradual step down the shoe spectrum.

Another factor is your running history. If you've been running for only a few years and did well on the tests, you can probably handle a bigger jump down than someone who's been running for 15 years in nothing but conventional training shoes. Your body won't have adapted as much as the veteran's to the altered mechanics caused by conventional running shoes. The rationale here is similar to most experts saying young runners can get away with running in less shoe because they're starting with a cleaner biomechanical slate, as we'll see in Chapter 8.

Also consider your typical training. If you do almost no hard workouts or races, where your feet and lower legs work through a fuller range of motion and generate more force, you're probably not ready for as minimal a shoe as someone who regularly does faster running. Similarly, if you're used to wearing racing flats or lightweight trainers for races and hard workouts, your Achilles, plantar fasciae, and calf muscles will be better prepared for a more minimal model than those of someone who wears more built-up training shoes for everything.

In terms of shoe features, focus on the ramp angle, or the difference in height from heel to forefoot. A good rule of thumb is to try a

WEIGHT FOR IT

In addition to your performance on these tests, consider your weight when deciding how aggressively to transition to minimalism. Experts like Jay Johnson, who offers online coaching advice for Nike, and Phil Wharton agree that if you're not at a good running weight, you should take a more conservative approach while working to get your weight down. As Wharton says, "If you're not at your optimal weight, there's so much extra stress on the joints, the 26 bones in the foot, all those little muscles down there."

minimalist shoe with a ramp angle that's about half that of your current model. To take just one example, say you know you like Asics, and have been in a traditional model like their Gel DS Trainer. It has a reported 10-millimeter heel-to-toe drop. You could try their Asics Gel Hyperspeed, which has a reported 5-millimeter heel-to-toe drop.

Of course, it's possible to pull off a greater jump in ramp angle. In those cases, walk before you run to see how conservative a transition you should attempt. "If you're gung-ho on going right to something like the FiveFingers, spend a day walking around in your new shoes," says coach Jay Johnson. "For a lot of people, your feet are going to get sore afterward. That'll give you an idea how much strength they need for you to run well in them."

A CONSERVATIVE TRANSITION PLAN

For almost everyone transitioning to minimalism, slower will get you there faster. Gradually integrating minimal shoes into your running will allow your body to adapt to the new stresses better than plunging right in. A month into the transition, you might not be running as much as you'd like in your new shoes, but 3 months in, you're more likely to still be progressing, and running healthfully and happily, than if you switch over too quickly. What's the rush? You have the rest of your running life to make the transition.

What constitutes a gradual transition is going to vary by runner. There are so many factors that will affect how you respond to running in minimalist shoes, including your strength and flexibility, running history, mileage, injury history, running surface, and more. This is definitely an area where the adage "we're all an experiment of one" is true. Consider the following strategies while conducting your experiment:

- **Start by walking.** This is something you can do from day 1. Wear your new minimalist shoes as daily footwear, as your professional responsibilities allow. The impact forces of walking are about one-third those of running, so your risk of injury is next to nothing. Spending a week walking in minimalist shoes will prepare your feet and lower legs for when you start running in them.

- **Go barefoot around the house.** Why wear shoes inside? Strengthen your feet and keep the floor clean at the same time! This is a good habit to stay in for the rest of your running life, regardless of what shoe you run in, because of the foot-strengthening benefits it provides.

- **When you start running in minimalist shoes, wear them at most every other day for the first 2 to 3 weeks.** "Fascia takes 48 hours to recover," says Wharton. Fascia is connective tissue that envelops muscles, bones, nerves, blood vessels, and organs. Among other roles, healthy fascia enables smooth movement of muscles by reducing friction. Tight fascia inhibits good running form and can lead to compensatory imbalances. You don't want overly tight fascia at any time in your running career, but especially when you're adding the new stress of running in minimalist shoes.

- **Start with just a mile or two at a time.** Logistically, this can be accomplished in a couple of ways. You can do the bulk of your run in your old shoes and wind up back at your starting point with a mile or two to go. Then change into your minimalist shoes for the remainder of the day's mileage. If you do workouts involving a warmup and cooldown, you could start by wearing them for one or both of those bookends, says Fullem.

- **Consider striders.** Striders (fast but relaxed runs of about 100 meters at the pace you can hold for a mile) are an essential part of most competitive runners' training. They help to build and maintain basic speed and are a great opportunity once or twice a week to concentrate on good running form. Wearing minimalist shoes for striders after an easy run helps you get used to the shoes in small doses while neurologically associating the shoes with good running form from the start.

- **Increase on a weekly, not per-run with basis.** Whatever amount of running you start, in your new shoes, hold at that level for at least a week. Then increase the next week only by whatever your original amount was. For example, if in the first week you ran in minimalist shoes for a mile at a time, go up to no more than 2 miles at a time the second week, 3 miles at a time the third week, and so on. Eventually you'll reach a time or mileage amount in your minimalist shoes that's at the low end of your range of regular runs, such as an easy 4-miler the day before your weekly long run.

- **Gradually integrate minimalist shoes into harder running.** If you regularly do track sessions, tempo runs, and other types of faster running, and don't already wear racing flats for these workouts, take the same conservative approach here as with mileage. If you're doing a track workout, you could quickly change shoes before the last one or two repeats. If it's a tempo day, you could break the tempo run into two or three segments with just enough rest between to change shoes. If you're doing a hill workout, you could put on your minimalist shoes for the last few charges uphill. Then, as with mileage, gradually increase the number of repeats or total amount of time spent running hard in minimalist shoes.

• **Always be ready to take a step back.** "If at any point you feel some discomfort that's beyond your muscles being sore, back off," says Peter Larson, author of the popular minimalist blog Runblogger. If you're an experienced runner, you probably know how to distinguish between acceptable niggles and pain that merits attention. Most muscular soreness should get better with gentle running. If you have a transition-related ache that doesn't improve once you're warmed up, then stop running in your minimalist shoes. Return to your regular shoes until the pain goes away, and start again from scratch.

A RADICAL TRANSITION PLAN

The above conservative transition plan is for the vast majority of runners. A more radical mode is that advocated by Mark

Cucuzzella, MD, owner of a minimalism-focused store in Shepherdstown, West Virginia. This plan entails immediately doing all your running in minimalist shoes but starting with, well, minimal mileage, such as a mile at a time. From there you gradually build to 2 miles per run, then 3 miles, and so on, until you're back to your normal mileage in a few months. In common with the conservative transition plan, here you also spend as much of your nonrunning time as possible barefoot or in zero-drop casual shoes.

This more extreme program makes the most sense for more desperate runners. It's what 2:37 marathoner Camille Herron, whom we met in Chapter 2, did after suffering seven stress fractures in a few years. The thinking here is that if you're chronically injured in regular running shoes, you need a more dramatic change in your routine. Once you're over your latest injury and are ready to resume running, make minimalist shoes an integral part of your new running life from the get-go, Cucuzzella advises. Of course, you don't have to be returning from injury to take this approach, but few healthy runners are willing to go cold turkey on mileage simply for the sake of adapting to new shoes.

Counterintuitive though it might seem, the best shoe for this approach is often a more minimal model than when transitioning gradually. You're essentially starting your running program from scratch. So your mileage will be quite low for some time, and your body should be able to handle the small amount of running you're doing even in a zero-drop, minimally cushioned model. With that safety factor built in, it makes sense to attempt to rewire your running mechanics in a shoe that allows for the most natural gait.

COMMON INJURIES WHILE TRANSITIONING TO MINIMALISM

Most runners are going to feel muscular aches in the early days of their transition to minimalist shoes. Unfortunately, some will experience more acute injuries, despite carrying out what seemed like a conservative plan. As Wharton explains, those minimalism-specific injuries are predictably from the knee down.

"As the heel has to drop, you're going to utilize a lot more of the calf unit, the gastrocnemius and soleus," he says, "and you're stretching the Achilles a little bit more, which is great long-term, but at the beginning it's really tough because you're not getting help from other muscles in close proximity on the kinetic chain. There's a lot more responsibility on these lower-leg muscles. So we get a lot of posterior tibial problems, tendinitis and ligament strains, peroneal tendon pain, even fractures."

Here are the three most common injuries runners encounter while transitioning to minimalist shoes, and what to do about them. In all these situations, once you have the acute phase under control, reboot your transition to minimalism by starting from scratch instead of diving back into where you were when you got injured.

Plantar Fasciitis

The plantar fascia is a thick, fibrous band of connective tissue that supports the arch. Running in a shoe with a lower heel and running with more of a midfoot strike require the plantar fascia to absorb more impact forces. "The arch was designed as a spring, and if that

BUILD YOUR RUNNING BODY

During your transition—and for the rest of your running life, for that matter—be dedicated about maintaining and increasing functional strength and flexibility. Regardless of how you performed on the five tests earlier in this chapter, do the "fix" exercise from each test a couple times a week. In addition, see "The Minimalist's Maintenance Tool Kit" in Chapter 8 for a series of simple but highly effective exercises you can do anywhere to stay a healthy minimalist runner.

spring isn't strong and flexible, then you're not going to be able to translate the shock of running to a specific mechanical change," says Wharton. Many runners have tight, weak plantar fasciae from decades of wearing shoes with heels, both while running and in daily life. A dramatic increase in the plantar fascia's workload can lead to almost immediate injury.

You'll feel a sharp, tearing pain along the inside bottom of your foot anywhere from the heel through the arch. Many times, the pain is the worst when you step out of bed in the morning or when you've been sitting for a long time; it tends to lessen with mild activity but then be present after you run.

You can usually run through plantar fasciitis, but you need to protect the fascia while it's inflamed. That means returning to conventional shoes until the pain subsides. Rolling your foot along a glass bottle you keep in the freezer provides a simultaneous icing and massage. Anti-inflammatories such as ibuprofen can also help to calm the fascia.

Achilles Tendinitis

The Achilles tendon is key to running with a midfoot landing and push-off. Like the plantar fascia, in most modern runners the Achillies has been shortened and weakened by elevated shoes for run-

MEET A MINIMALIST

ADRIENNE LEIGH MENDENHALL
SINGAPORE

An American living in the city-state of Singapore, Adrienne Leigh Mendenhall notes, "There is definitely a strong following for Vibram [FiveFingers] over here, both on roads and trails." She hopes to eventually be one of the Singapore runners wearing them, but is working toward that goal gradually after her first go-round with the shoes was too sudden and led to setbacks.

Mendenhall began running as a high school student in the mid-1990s. She wore conventional shoes, usually beefy models like the Asics Kayano, for the next 15 years. After reading *Born to Run*, in 2010 she bought a pair of FiveFingers in the hope that they would help with hip and knee pain that had been plaguing her for years. Although she's a marathon

veteran, including in the soupy climate of Singapore, Mendenhall's main motivation is to be able to run for years. She thought a switch to Vibrams would help.

"I started out slow, with 1 mile at a time," she says, "built up to 7-mile runs with a tiny bit of fifth metatarsal pain, but figured if the pain didn't get worse, then it would eventually get better. Smart? No. Typical impatience of a runner? Yes."

At the time, she was living in Minnesota, and one icy night she opted for the treadmill. Figuring that the need for the slight surficial protection that Vibram provides on roads wasn't needed on the treadmill, she ran barefoot. As Mendenhall puts it, "Inaugural barefoot running plus treadmill boredom—playing with speed ning, work, and leisure. So, like the plantar fascia, it's easily overloaded if you suddenly start running in shoes with a minimal ramp angle. Bloodflow to the tendon is relatively poor; the tendon is slower to warm up than some other key running body parts.

and incline—equals ouch." She had strained a tendon or ligament in her already-hurting foot. "So, we can chalk up the next 2 months of sedentary wistfulness to stupidity," she says.

When Mendenhall's foot got better, she returned to conventional Asics, the 2150, and, she says, "decided to approach minimalist running with a logical plan. I've been stepping down the cushioning in each pair of running shoes." From the Asics 2150 she went to the Brooks PureFlow while using the Asics Sky Speed for long runs. About the latter, she says, "Frankly, I detest their weight and bulk, but I'm still hesitant about lightweight shoes and the potential for injury if my feet and ankles aren't ready."

Then Mendenhall bought the Merrell Pace Glove and began to work them into her training conservatively, starting with just a few 3-milers. "I'll slowly add distance to these short runs until they equal the distance of a normal run," she says. If as she adapts she feels like the difference between the fairly cushioned Brooks and barely there Merrell is too great, she's open to a shoe that lies between the two to aid the transition.

And what about those FiveFingers so many others in Singapore run in? "I haven't put them on for over a year but am getting antsy to give them another shot," Mendenhall says. "I liked running in them before, and the goal is to eventually run regularly in them again. But first I need to be pain-free."

Like plantar fasciitis, Achilles tendinitis produces a sharp, tugging sensation, in this case from the back of your heel up to the bottom of your calf muscles. In severe cases, you'll be able to see swelling. Unlike with plantar fasciitis, the pain tends to get worse, not better, with running.

Icing and anti-inflammatories can help to reduce the inflammation. Mild stretching—never to the point of producing pain—can help increase bloodflow to the tendon. You can try to run through Achilles tendinitis in your conventional shoes, but unless you want it to drag on forever, you'll need to lower your mileage dramatically, do nothing but run slowly, and avoid hills as much as possible. If the tendon is so aggravated that it's noticeably larger than your healthy one, you're usually better off not running until you get the most severe inflammation under control.

Metatarsal Stress Fractures and Stress Reactions

Running in minimalist shoes often reveals underlying weaknesses throughout the body. In many runners, says Wharton, "a lot of the muscles that are supposed to be doing their job, like the glutes, hamstrings, hip rotators, and iliopsoas, aren't doing their jobs. This tends to lead to a harder footplant." Conventional running shoes tend to accommodate this form flaw better than minimalist shoes, thanks to plush cushioning. With less material between you and the ground, running in minimalist shoes puts more of the impact force from bad form on the bones of your feet, especially the metatarsals, the five long bones running from midfoot to the base of the toes.

Stress reactions are precursors to stress fractures. Initially you'll feel a dull ache over a small area in the front or middle of your foot.

As with most stress reactions and fractures, pressing on the sore spot will likely cause pinpoint pain. Although you may have heard that you can't run on a stress fracture, we runners are a tough, dedicated bunch, and it's possible to run on a fractured foot, at your normal mileage, no matter how ill-advised doing so is. If the pain is worse after you run, then you're well along the path of a stress reaction becoming a full-blown fracture.

Although you can run on a stress fracture, you shouldn't. There's no finessing your way through the process of getting a weight-bearing bone to heal. Metatarsal stress fractures usually require 1 to 2 months of no running for proper healing. If you've caught the problem early (you can produce pinpoint pain by pressing, you feel it when you run, but it's not worse hours after a run), then you can get away with less time off. But as with transitioning to minimalist shoes, a little more conservatism in the short run can lead to fewer setbacks a couple of months down the road.

How Low Should You Go?

Let's say you've successfully transitioned from a conventional training shoe into one of the gateway minimalist models like the Saucony Kinvara, or even something more minimal. Should you keep moving through the minimalist spectrum to a lighter, lower shoe? Should everyone's goal be running solely in barely there shoes or barefoot?

As with so much in running, there are no universal answers here. Start by remembering that minimalist shoes are a means to the goal of better running form. They're part of a tool kit that, ideally, also includes core strength and functional flexibility, training at a variety of paces and being at a good running weight, and other factors that contribute to being a healthy, efficient runner. We can all run with better form in whatever shoes we have. Focusing only on the ramp angle and stack height of your shoes is, frankly, being irresponsible. "You can't just get to a certain point and say, 'Okay, I've got these shoes that are a 6-millimeter drop, I'm running a little better, but I just don't feel like doing drills anymore,'" says Brian Metzler, coauthor of *Natural Running*. "You've got to keep it up and do everything across the board."

Minimalist blogger Larson says, "I wouldn't say, 'You're in the Kinvara now, so you have to go down to something like the New Balance 1600 [a light racing flat].' I think that's what some people do. They feel like, 'I have to continue this progression until I'm running in nothing.'

"That doesn't have to be the end point. When the Kinvara came out, I was talking with one of the guys from Saucony, and he was telling me they have this internal debate about that—what do you tell people? Is this an end-point shoe or a gateway shoe? My response is it could be either. You need to decide that for yourself.

"Initially my own goal was 'Maybe I should be doing all my running in something like the Vibram FiveFingers,'" Larson continues. "I've come back to the realization that wearing a shoe with a little bit of cushioning is not an evil thing if it allows you to run the way you want to run."

That last point is key. Just as there are other aspects of running with good form than your shoes, there are other aspects of running than your form. "Of course running form is important," says Joe Rubio, who coaches several national-class runners in California.

"But to think about it all the time . . . sometimes you just want to go for a run, you know?"

"That's especially true on the trails," says Metzler, who was the founding editor of *Trail Runner* magazine. "Depending on the trails and shoes, you can run as nimbly as possible but still feel every pebble, stalk, or notch on the trail. To go through a whole run like that isn't always the most enjoyable thing to do.

"But even on the roads, there are a lot of obstacles out there, whether it's stepping off a curb or on a pebble," Metzler continues. "Do you want to have every step of the way be this aware, eyes-on-the-road thing, or do you just want to run and zone out? I think for most runners there's a happy medium where you're in a shoe that promotes good form but also offers enough protection so that most days you're just running and not thinking about your shoes and form the whole way."

If, for most runners, the transition to minimalist shoes doesn't necessarily mean running in as little as possible, where does that leave barefoot running? Is there a role for running without shoes in most runners' programs? The answer is yes, and that's the subject of the next chapter.

7

REASONABLE BAREFOOTING

The theory and practice of running without shoes

ONE DAY IN THE EARLY 1980s, I found myself at my sister's house without running gear. For reasons I can't recall, there was only this window of time that day when I'd be able to run. So I borrowed a T-shirt and pair of tennis shorts from my sister and ran barefoot on the roads for an hour. I remember getting stares.

Whether that was because of the lack of shoes on asphalt or the women's tennis shorts, I can't say. Certainly I was an anomaly.

The thing is, I would be an anomaly today as well, even in the most staid running attire. For all you hear about barefoot running, few runners regularly do it.

That's a shame. Running barefoot has many benefits, including simply feeling good when you can find a suitable surface. In Chapter 4, we saw how most runners who are used to going unshod adopt a midfoot strike, compared with the heel strike most runners in shoes use, and that barefoot runners don't overstride as often as shod runners do. We also saw that most runners have better running economy when barefoot.

This chapter is about the intersection of barefoot running theory and modern running. We'll start by looking at an elegant hypothesis by Harvard anthropologist Daniel Lieberman on the role of (barefoot) running in human evolution, then move on to practical recommendations for regularly adding barefoot running to your training.

THE RUNNING MAN THEORY

If you've read *Born to Run,* or even read about *Born to Run,* you know that Lieberman thinks that running was central to our species' development. Call it the Running Man theory. Briefly stated, it goes like this.

Humans are better than other mammals at dissipating heat. Running in the heat of the day, our African ancestors were able to chase game until the prey collapsed. Because the most successful subsistence hunters were the most likely to survive and pass on their genes, natural selection favored proficiency in long-distance running. At the same time, the meat from the animals provided enough high-quality protein to stimulate brain growth, which further separated humans from other primates. The next thing you know, humans had spread throughout the world and invented the Internet, where people can spend all day debating what shoes to run in. Running helped to make us human.

The news-you-can-use corollary to the main theory is that most of this running occurred barefoot on hard, uneven surfaces. Even once humans started running in footwear, it was minimal footwear, from the Paleolithic Era of 45,000 years ago until the invention of the modern running shoe in the 1970s. So humans must be well adapted to running long distances barefoot. Modern running shoes are the aberration; running barefoot is the default. The form that humans use when running barefoot is the natural way to run and will lead to less injury, proponents say. The best way to run with that form, obviously, is to run barefoot.

SOME "YEAH, BUT . . ." THOUGHTS

The evolutionary part of the Running Man theory is wonderful. We've all had runs when everything's clicking and we feel the elemental rightness of what we're doing. And of course it's flattering to hear our beloved sport posited as integral to human progress.

Lieberman, who does a lot of his running barefoot, hasn't said the Running Man theory means everyone should run barefoot. Others have, and hold up Running Man as the ideal to which all runners should aspire. Here are a few points to consider about how Running Man might differ from his 21st-century counterparts.

Evolution continues. Modern humans are thought to have started branching out from Africa 125,000 years ago. UCLA professor Jared Diamond, author of the 1997 bestseller *Gun, Germs, and Steel,* notes that food production began to replace the hunter-gatherer mode of existence 11,000 years ago. These are, of course, blips on the timeline of human evolution over a couple of million years. But whatever evolutionary selection may have once occurred in favor of barefoot running, it hasn't been nearly as significant in most of the world for hundreds of generations now. Human evolution didn't stop at some random date in the past; natural selection has favored traits other than running aptitude, in environments other than the African savanna, for quite a while now.

Experiment of one. When Running Man adherents wonder about injury rates, that seems partly based on the notion that we should all be able to run without getting hurt. But we have no way of knowing how often Running Man was injured, nor do we know if everyone was a regular hunter. Perhaps only the Mo Farahs of the day were sent out to hunt, and as the meat providers, they had the highest status and most often passed along their genes. (The best distance runners having alpha status—talk about differences with modern runners!)

There's a difference between what the species has evolved to do and what any one member of the species is capable of. It's pretty easy to think of ways in which aptitude in spatial relations would have an evolutionary advantage, yet you're reading a book written by someone who didn't learn to tie his shoes until third grade. Running with good mechanics is another evolved trait that some individuals lack. That should be increasingly true over time when that trait is no longer being worked on by natural selection.

Gender of the runner. Although we don't have demographic info on the Great Antelope Hunt 10-Miler of 20,000 BC, it's logical to think that all or nearly all the participants were men. (Young men, for that matter. More on that in a bit.) In 2011, 53 percent of finishers in US half-marathons were women. This is as it should be. But women have wider pelvises and less muscle than men and can have different running mechanics.

Age of the runner. How to spend his senior years wasn't a pressing issue for Running Man. Skeletal evidence from Neanderthal times through the beginning of the Common Era (i.e., what we call year 0) indicates that the mean human life span was about 30 years. The median age of today's *Runner's World* subscriber is 41. People in their 80s regularly finish marathons. With age come physiological changes, such as loss of muscle mass, that can affect one's running mechanics.

History of the runner. In Running Man days, running would have been a regular part of one's life soon after becoming bipedal. Many modern runners do the first half-hour run of their life in their 30s, 40s, or older. This is quite different from the state that the Running Man theory suggests is the default human condition.

Size of the runner. Even as recently as the late 19th century, the average American looked different than today. The average Union soldier in the Civil War is estimated to have stood 5'8" and weighed

143 pounds. Running Man was almost certainly smaller than that. Sport podiatrist Kevin Kirby says, "When the average adult male runner now weighs 185 pounds versus probably the average male weight of 125 pounds thousands of years ago, the injury rates during running will naturally increase, regardless if they were barefoot or in shoes. This seems so obvious to me both from a biomechanical modeling aspect and from my experience as a clinician, but none of

MEET A MINIMALIST

GREG DIAMOND
CORTLANDT MANOR, NEW YORK

Greg Diamond is a great example of a longtime runner who's worked principles of minimalism into an established, successful running program. Now in his mid-50s, he's running faster on an age-graded basis than he was 15 years ago. A few years ago, he was the New York Road Runners Runner of the Year in the 50-to-54 age group. He credits part of that accomplishment to running more in less shoe, supplemented by small doses of barefoot running.

Diamond started doing short barefoot stints simply because "it just sounded right to me," he says. "I believe that we have weakened our feet with footwear." He began

extremely conservatively, running just a 10th of a mile on a treadmill the first time, and increasing by another 10th of a mile every other run. "I knew that doing it very gradually had to be the only way," he says. "I knew better than to run a mile first time out."

These days he does about 4 miles a week on the treadmill—some barefoot, the rest in the ZEMgear Ninja Split Toe High, a 2.3-ounce, slipperlike, ankle-high shoe that provides him abrasion protection on the moving belt of the treadmill. ("I tried the Vibram FiveFingers, an early version, and found them too clunky," he says.) He also runs in one of the lightest racing flats on the market, the Mizuno Wave Universe, and the barefoot advocates tend to mention body weight as being a very significant factor in injury production."

Road versus savanna. An obvious and almost always immediate objection to the Running Man theory is some form of "Our ancestors didn't evolve running on asphalt." True, but that doesn't necessarily scuttle the theory. Lieberman likes to point out that the savanna on which Running Man did his running was hard, not soft like grass or

has worn the Saucony Kinvara for lots of long runs and a marathon. In all, Diamond estimates that he does 20 to 35 percent of his mileage, which can get as high as 100 a week, barefoot or in minimalist shoes.

Although Diamond started his barefoot experiment for its own sake, "I realized how strong my feet were becoming, how I was switching to forefoot/midfoot strike even in regular shoes, how this was translating into less lower-leg soreness in races," he says. "Now my major motivation is to keep my feet strong and my stride healthy as I get older. I ran a half-marathon in the Mizuno Wave Universe with no soreness at all. I remember running a half-marathon in a shoe twice as heavy at 41 and barely walking away from it. It is so amazing to me that I can run all these hard miles in 3.5-ounce shoes with no cushioning."

Diamond's transition was eased by years of good habits in his nonrunning hours. "I have always walked around barefoot or in socks," he says. (His wife calls his practice "socks as shoes.") Also, as a longtime competitive runner—he ran a 2:41 marathon in 1995—he was used to running in racing flats. So his feet and lower legs were stronger than average and readier than most people's when he shifted to more minimalist and barefoot running.

sand. We should also keep in mind the fascinating finding from Chapter 4 that we make adjustments to account for the firmness of the surface we're running on.

At the same time, it should be noted that Lieberman's assessment of the ancestral running surface is based on his time running in Africa, not durometer readings of ancient soil. Like most of the longtime Western runners who've run in Kenya, I think modern American roads are harder than the African earth. (I'm not counting Kenya's clay roads, which obviously didn't exist in Running Man's time.) I did barefoot striders on random Kenyan ground with what felt like normal mechanics. If I were to do them on my street, I would run them with slightly different form. Running comfortably and injury-free on asphalt is eventually within most people's capacity, but it will probably look a little different than running barefoot on a natural surface. And this leads us to perhaps the major caveat concerning the Running Man theory.

Ancient versus modern running. Running as would have occurred in the evolutionary setting is significantly different from the running that most of us do. Running Man didn't do track workouts early in the morning before heading off to work. He no doubt ran long and fast at times, but he ran only when he had to, and only as long and hard as was necessary. He didn't follow 16-week schedules leading up to a marathon. Put another way, running is a natural activity. Training to run 26.2 miles as fast as you can on the roads, not so much. The Running Man theory asks why so many people get injured despite what variables are present in their running. Training for excellence is a variable that seems an obvious means of injury.

As for Running Man and racing, he didn't do it like we do. In terms of mechanics, remember from Chapter 4 that most runners shorten their stride and increase their turnover when they go from shod to barefoot. For well-trained runners, this could be a performance limiter at faster speeds. When you run markedly faster than your normal training pace, your turnover increases. At some point you'll bump up against the upper limit of cadence you can sustain for the duration of a race. If, at the same time, you're doing something (running barefoot) that shortens your stride length, then you won't be running as fast as you could. When asked about barefoot running, two-time Olympic marathoner Ryan Hall has said, "The best guys in the world are wearing shoes and we're running fast. [When] some barefoot dude comes by me at 26 miles, then maybe I'll look into it."

If the Running Man theory inspires you to explore daily barefoot running, go for it. But don't feel subhuman if you decide to wear something on your feet for most of your runs.

Best Uses of Barefoot Running

I could go out today and, more than 30 years after doing so from my sister's house, run for an hour barefoot on the roads with no issues. I just don't want to. For me, watching every step for pebbles or glass or other common features of American roads detracts from enjoying the run.

You, of course, should do what you want in this regard. You'll quickly learn your preferences for where—or whether—to do everyday runs barefoot, and in what range of conditions. Here in

Maine, I've run barefoot on grass as early in the year as March and as late as November. There's a regular barefoot-on-roads runner in my area whom I've seen running in December. There's great variability in runners' tolerance for cold, and that includes when running barefoot.

But let's step back and assume that, like most people, you haven't run barefoot in a long time. What's the best way to get started?

Begin by keeping in mind the overall message of my nitpicky points from above about the Running Man theory. Modern runners are fairly far removed from the ancestral setting. As sport scientist Ross Tucker puts it, injury-free barefoot running should be considered a skill. As with all skills, some will acquire it almost immediately, many will acquire it with more practice, and some might never acquire it. (The last group might be those who heel-strike when running barefoot and overload the plantar area.) Whatever caution you may exercise when moving from conventional running shoes to minimalist models, be even more conservative when you start experimenting with barefoot running.

Your first barefoot runs should be quite short, in the neighborhood of 5 minutes of easy running. Logistically, you could do this by

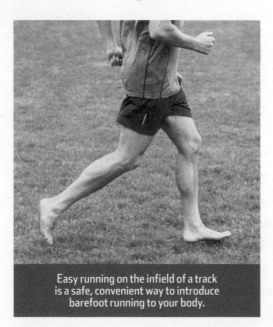

Easy running on the infield of a track is a safe, convenient way to introduce barefoot running to your body.

starting your run from a playing field, heading out on the roads for the bulk of your run, then returning to your starting point and shedding your shoes for the last few minutes. Because there's such great variance in acquiring the skill of barefoot running, universal rules aren't possible. But again, err on the side of caution. Give yourself a few days to a week until you try again. Add in small increments—think minutes, not miles. Respect the difference between a little tenderness the day after and pain during or after.

Cooldowns and More

If you do regular track workouts, experiment with doing some of your cooldown barefoot on the interior of the track. Elite coach Steve Magness says, "I like the barefoot cooldown as a way to introduce barefoot running. It's going to be a little lower impact because you're going pretty slow after a workout. It's an easy conditioning and strengthening tool for the feet."

Jay Johnson, who used to coach a group of national-class runners in Boulder, Colorado, also favors barefoot cooldowns. "They all loved the sensation of running barefoot after track workouts," he says about his former runners, who included national champions in indoor track and cross-country. "We would do 10 laps of the interior of the field, which is basically 2 miles of running. They really felt like it strengthened their feet and lower legs, and I think, most importantly, they liked how it feels."

Another common use of barefoot running is strides. If you enjoy easy barefoot running on natural surfaces and want to try to further strengthen your feet, consider barefoot strides on an unrutted field or the interior of the track. Here the logistics would be similar

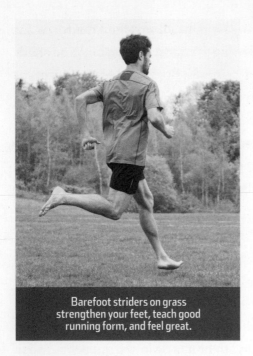

Barefoot striders on grass strengthen your feet, teach good running form, and feel great.

to ending a run with easy barefoot running. Finish a regular easy-to-moderate run at a place where you can safely and comfortably run barefoot, and do 8 to 10 100-meter strides at mile race-pace effort.

"I think the best use for barefoot running is strengthening the arch with strides," says physiotherapist Phil Wharton. "Easy barefoot running, like in a cooldown, is the starting point and segue. But there's nothing like barefoot strides if you can find a great grass surface. It really does help rebuild the feet. Afterward it can be almost the same feeling you get when you do a whole session of foot/ankle towel curls and ankle inversion/eversion exercises with a weighted sock. You can just feel that lever strengthening." (We'll learn all about towel curls and weighted-sock exercises in the next chapter.)

Magness has another use for barefoot strides. "I like them as a feedback mechanism if you're working on form," he says. "Take the shoes off, do some strides, throw the shoes back on and do some strides and you say, 'Oh, okay, there is a difference.' It's a feedback cue. You get the sensation of what it feels like barefoot and then try to recall that on other runs."

As Magness points out, you can't accumulate as much volume of barefoot running doing strides as you can in a cooldown. As you continue to adapt to barefoot running, you can get good barefoot volume and strengthening benefits by doing a Kenyan specialty called diagonals.

A session of diagonals consists of mixing strides and jogging. Envision a rectangular grass surface such as a football field. When doing diagonals, you jog from one end of the goal line to the other, then run fast from that corner to the opposite corner of the other goal line. Then you jog to the end of that goal line, and then run fast from that corner to where you started jogging on the other goal line. Your path will have made an X across the interior of the field, plus solid lines at the top and bottom of the X. For most runners, it will take roughly as long to run fast diagonally across the field as it will to jog from one end of the goal line to the other.

Everyone in Kenya, from milers to marathoners, does diagonals. They're fun, short workouts that help build basic speed and smooth out your running form. Doing them barefoot adds a foot-strengthening aspect. Do diagonals in units of time, not repeats, so that you can concentrate on good running form rather than how many times you've crisscrossed the field. Start with 5 or 10 minutes. That's plenty of time to get the benefits. If you come to enjoy diagonals, consider making the sessions longer and treating them like fartlek sessions that replace a harder workout in your schedule.

A few years ago, Halloween was freakishly warm in Maine. I knew how best to savor the day—I headed to the waterside field where I do diagonals. For 40 minutes I strode and jogged barefoot while the sun set over the Casco Bay. For that brief time, I felt like

Running Man. And if you ever want to feel the difference between running barefoot and in shoes, do 40 minutes of barefoot diagonals and then put on your trainers for a 15-minute run home.

Small bits of regular barefoot running can safely and enjoyably become part of most runners' lifelong programs. What else to do to be a healthy, happy minimalist for the rest of your running life is the subject of the next chapter.

CHAPTER 8

MINIMALISM
FOR LIFE

How to stay healthy long-term
while running in less shoe

ALMOST ALL RUNNERS hope to run for the rest of their lives and to never be injured while doing so. Working toward that ideal is probably your main motivation for running in minimalist shoes. This chapter is about what you can do to marry minimalism with a lifetime of running.

First we'll see how to do some key exercises that help you run with good form in any shoes, but especially in minimalist shoes. Then we'll learn a few drills that will help hardwire improved form into your daily runs. We'll see what to do when not running to best preserve your running body, and consider whether minimalism is right for runners of all ages. We'll end by addressing this question: Should you commit to doing every run for the rest of your life in minimalist shoes?

THE MINIMALIST'S MAINTENANCE TOOL KIT

"If you want to become a better runner, begin by running better," says Pete Magill, a California coach and the oldest American to break 15:00 for 5-K, which he did a few months before his 50th birthday.

By that Magill means doing things that improve your ability to run more efficiently and with good form. Learning to run well in minimalist shoes is one means toward that goal. But for almost all runners, switching shoes isn't sufficient. Typical Western lifestyles, with lots of time spent sitting and little time spent doing a wide variety of activities that work the whole body through a variety of motions, make many of the muscles needed to run with good form weak and tight.

Put another way, all modern runners should consider regular bodywork integral to their running, not something only elites who have all day to train or people returning from injury do. Consider strengthening key running-specific muscles as both a performance enhancer and a form of insurance. "Any runner, no matter what shoe they wear, if they want to do one thing to try to prevent injury, I would recommend targeted strengthening," says sport podiatrist Brian Fullem.

Minimalist runners are especially good candidates for this work. As we saw in Chapter 6, weakness and/or tightness in key lower-leg muscles and your core can increase your risk of injury when you start running in minimalist shoes. What you need in these areas is functional strength and mobility—that is, strength and mobility to meet the specific demands of maintaining good running form and being resistant to injury. "Sorry, but these aren't your beach muscles," says physiotherapist Phil Wharton. "A lot of them are tiny muscles no one's ever going to see, but that absolutely need to be functioning to run with good form in minimalist shoes."

Although we tend to focus on the lower legs when we talk about the requirements of running in minimalist shoes, core strength—in your hips, glutes, lower back, and abdomen—is vital. Good core strength will help you maintain a stable pelvic position while running, saving your lower legs from getting overloaded by the impact forces of running. If you notice that you start runs with good form when wearing minimalist shoes but then get sloppy after a few miles, that's an indication that you need to improve your core strength.

The following exercises strengthen and improve flexibility in the key running muscles in your feet, legs, and core that contribute to good running form. Do this group of exercises at least twice and preferably three times a week. The whole set won't take you longer than 15 minutes and makes for a nice postrun routine. If you're motivated to go beyond the exercises here, Wharton (whartonper formance.com) and coach Jay Johnson (runningdvds.com) have excellent, extensive resources in the form of books, DVDs, and short instructional videos.

WEIGHTED-SOCK SWING

Weighted-sock swings build lower-leg and foot strength.

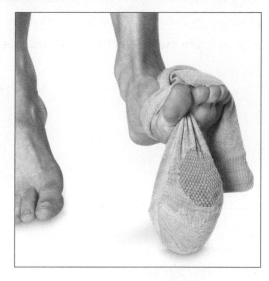

Why: This exercise strengthens your lower-leg muscles and the muscles that support and form your arch.

How: Stuff a 1- or 2-pound weight into the toe of a long sock. (Finally, a nonembarrassing use for compression socks!) Place the sock between your big toe and second toe with the weight dangling under the ball of your foot. Make a stirrup by wrapping the end of the sock around the outside of your foot, under your arch, and back up over the top of your foot. Fasten it securely by tying under the top wrap.

Sit on a high enough surface so that the weighted sock doesn't touch the floor, with your back straight, your knees slightly apart, and your lower legs dangling. Point your foot down so that your big toe is pointing at the floor. Sweep your foot up and toward the midline of your body, pointing your big toe to the ceiling. Pause, then sweep your foot back down to the starting position, with your big toe pointing straight down at the floor.

Without pausing, sweep your foot up and away from your body as far as possible. Slowly return to the starting position. Imagine the full movement forming a U in the air. The whole pendulum sweep should take you about 8 to 10 seconds. Do 10 full sweeps (10 in each direction). Repeat on the other foot. Do two sets of 10 for each foot. (For convenience's sake, consider getting enough weights to have a weighted sock wrapped around each foot.)

Over time, you can add more weight to the socks. Don't add so much weight that the sweeping movement becomes strained. It should feel like a good assisted stretch, not a taxing weight-lifting movement.

SEATED CALF RAISE

Seated calf raises strengthen the soleus.

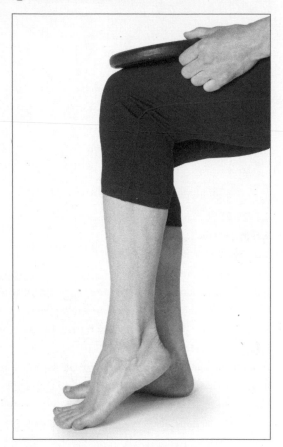

Why: This exercise strengthens your soleus, the calf muscle that's the main supplier of blood to your lower legs, ankles, and feet.

How: Sit with your legs bent at 90 degrees and your feet flat on the floor. Place a weight on top of one knee. The weight should be heavy enough so that you feel the soleus working when you do this exercise, but not so heavy that your calf is sore after. When in doubt, start with a lighter weight.

Keeping your toes on the floor and your knee bent at 90 degrees, raise your heel as far as you can by pushing up with your toes. Take 2 to 3 seconds to go up and another 2 to 3 seconds to come down. Do 10 reps, switch the weight to the other leg and do 10 reps, and then do another set of 10 reps with each leg.

Over time, add more weight.

TOWEL PULL

Towel pulls strengthen the arch.

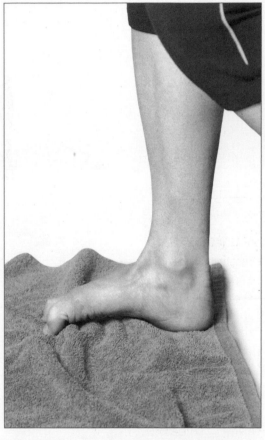

Why: This exercise strengthens your medial and lateral arch, especially the medial (inside) arch.

How: On a slick surface such as a wood or tile floor, place a towel so that the short end is in front of a chair you're sitting in. Sit straight with bare feet and with your legs bent at 90 degrees. Place your foot on the edge of the towel; throughout the exercise, keep your heel flat on the towel. Using only your foot muscles, reach out with your toes and contract them to grab a bit of the towel and pull it toward you. Concentrate on spreading your toes as you pull the towel toward you. Do 10 pulls, then straighten the towel to the starting position. Do another set of 10. Repeat with your other foot.

Once you've mastered regular towel pulls, make them more challenging by placing a small weight on the middle of the towel.

CLAM

Clams strengthen the glutes and hip rotators.

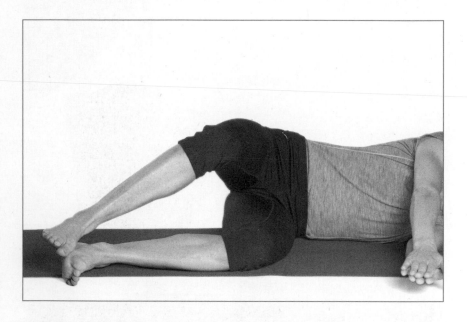

Why: This exercise strengthens your glutes and hip rotators. Better strength in these crucial core muscles will lessen common form flaws like splayed feet, an uneven pelvis, excessive lateral rotation, and leaning forward at the waist.

How: Lie on your left side with your legs together and bent at a 90-degree angle. Hold your arms together, extended in front of you. While keeping your feet together and your left leg on the floor, lift your right knee as if your legs were an open clamshell. Do the movement slowly—2 to 3 seconds going up, 2 to 3 seconds coming down—rather than rushing through as quickly as you can. Do 10 reps on that side, then switch sides and do 10 with the other leg.

Over time you can make the exercise more challenging by attaching a Theraband around your legs near the knees.

KNEE CIRCLE

Knee circles improve hip mobility.

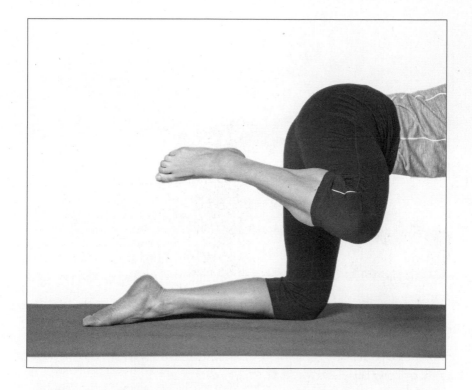

Why: This exercise will dramatically increase range of motion in your hip joints.

How: Start on your hands and knees on the floor, hands under your shoulders, knees under your hips. Keeping your right knee bent at 90 degrees, lift your right leg and lead with your knee moving forward to sweep the leg in a circular motion. Ideally your knee will come near your hip at the top of the circle. Do 10 forward circles, return to the starting position, and do 10 backward circles. Backward circles will probably be more challenging. Repeat with the other leg.

SIDE LEG RAISE

Side leg raises strengthen stabilizing muscles
in the hips and butt.

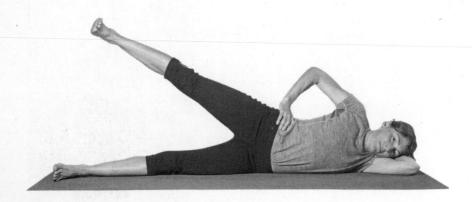

Why: In its three variations, this exercise strengthens the small stabilizing hip and
butt muscles, especially the gluteus medius.

How: Lie on your left side with your legs extended out straight. Your left arm
can rest under your head; your top arm can rest on your hip. With your right foot
parallel to your left foot, lift your right leg. Keep your hips steady and facing forward.
Lower the leg. Take 2 to 3 seconds to go up and 2 to 3 seconds to come down. Do
5 reps with your right foot in this neutral position. Then maintain the original position
except turn your right foot out so that the toes point toward the ceiling. Do 5 reps
in this position. Finally, maintain the original position except turn your right foot
in so that your toes point toward the floor. Do 5 reps in this position. (This last position will be the most challenging for most runners.) Do the same sequence of five
reps in each of the three foot positions with the other leg.

When you can do all three positions without your working leg shaking, make
the exercise more challenging by wearing ankle weights.

DONKEY KICK

Donkey kicks strengthen the glutes.

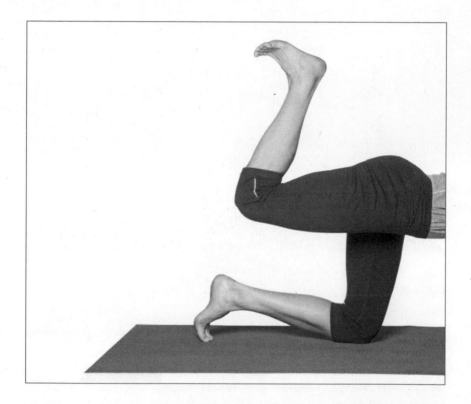

Why: This exercise strengthens your glutes, thereby enhancing your hip extension.

How: Start on your hands and knees on the floor, with your back straight but relaxed. Your hands should be under your shoulders, and your knees should be under your hips. Keeping your right knee bent, kick your right foot back and up so that the bottom of your foot faces the ceiling and then, without pausing, moves toward your back like a hook. Keeping your knee bent, return to the starting position and then move past it so that your knee nears your chest. Do 10 times with each leg.

PRONE PEDESTAL

The prone pedestal strengthens deep abdominal muscles.

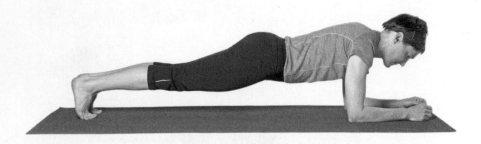

Why: This exercise strengthens your deep abdominal muscles. (You may have heard it and the other pedestal positions that follow called planks.)

How: Balance on your forearms and toes on the floor. Your elbows should be bent at 90 degrees and your toes should be slightly dorsiflexed (pointing up). Keep your shoulders, neck, and head stable but relaxed; don't scrunch up your shoulders or place all your weight on your elbows. Keep a straight line from your shoulders to your ankles. Concentrate on keeping your hips level, neither sagging toward the floor nor elevated so that your butt points up. Hold for 30 seconds.

Over time increase to holding for 60 seconds.

SUPINE PEDESTAL

The supine pedestal strengthens core muscles along the backside.

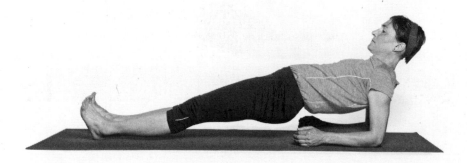

Why: This exercise strengthens your hamstrings, glutes, and lower-back muscles.

How: This is basically the flip side of the prone pedestal position. Balance on your elbows and heels, belly button pointing up. As with the prone pedestal, keep a straight line from your shoulders to your feet. Tuck your chin slightly toward your chest. Hold for 30 seconds.

Over time increase to holding for 60 seconds.

SIDE PEDESTAL

The side pedestal strengthens lower-back and abdominal muscles.

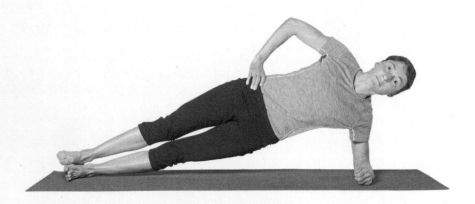

Why: This exercise strengthens your lower-back and side abdominal muscles.

How: Balance yourself on your left elbow and your feet, with the right foot stacked on top of the left foot. Place your right hand on your waist. Your left elbow should be under your left shoulder, with plenty of space between your left shoulder and head. Keep a straight line from your right shoulder to your feet. Don't allow your hips to drop. Hold for 30 seconds, then repeat on the other side.

There are several ways to make this exercise more challenging. First, increase to holding for 60 seconds. Then switch to balancing on your hand instead of your elbow. In that position, the closer you keep your top arm to your body, the more difficult the side pedestal will be. Finally, you can progress to doing side pedestals with your eyes closed.

Running Form Drills

Most elite runners do drills at least a couple of times a week. Most recreational runners don't. That's a shame, because devoting just a little time each week to these exercises has so many benefits—you'll recruit muscle fibers needed to run with your best form, correct muscle imbalances, become accustomed to moving through a fuller range of motion, and retrain your nervous system. These gains will help you run with better form at all speeds.

Runners moving to minimalist shoes are especially good candidates for drills. Remember, minimalist shoes are a means to the end of running more efficiently and effectively. Drills are another means toward that goal of improved form. Refining your running body with drills will make it easier to hold the improved form you're hoping to achieve by running in minimalist shoes.

Do drills at least once and preferably twice a week. When you're new to drills, do them after one of your easier runs of the week. As you get used to doing drills, you can do them pretty much any day. Many competitive runners include drills as part of their warmup before races and hard workouts, to help prime their bodies to operate at peak capacity.

You can do drills anywhere you have a flat, level surface for 30 to 50 yards—road, track, grass. Drills on a grass field feel good, but make sure there aren't divots or other hazards waiting to trip you up. In terms of convenience, your street is a great venue if it doesn't have a lot of traffic—you finish your run, do your drills, then head in for the day. And the neighbors will enjoy watching you.

There are an infinite number of drills you can do. The six that follow complement each other by working key aspects of having and holding the form you're trying to attain by running in minimalist shoes. If you'd like to learn more drills, I recommend DVDs put out (separately) by Johnson and another coach, Greg McMillan.

Do these drills in your minimalist shoes or barefoot. Complete each drill twice. Perform the drill as described, turn around and jog back to the starting point, then turn around again and run fast but relaxed over the same stretch. Adding that quick strideout (not a sprint!) after doing the drill will help to hardwire the movement pattern into your form. After doing the strideout, walk back to the starting point or walk around the area where you finished long enough so that you're suffi-

SHOSHANNA COHEN
PORTLAND, OREGON

Shoshanna Cohen's story is a good reminder that we're not just runners when we're running, but all day. Put another, perhaps less obsessive-sounding way, Cohen has learned the hard way that what we do in our nonrunning hours can have significant effects on our running.

Cohen began running in 2004, when she was in her mid-20s. In the fall of 2011, encouraged by the injury-prevention promises of minimalism, she gradually switched from conventional stability shoes to barely there Merrells, after a transition period of walking and standing in the Merrells while working retail. "Once I started, it just felt really good and was more fun than running in regular shoes, and that became my motivation, in addition to injury prevention," she says. "So much lighter and nimbler than the stability shoes, like going

from a station wagon to a sports car."

But then she apparently threw too much change at her body at once. "I got a pair of Vivobarefoot casual shoes to wear walking around town and starting wearing them everywhere," Cohen says. "I thought I'd be fine since I'd transitioned to Merrells already, but they were apparently different. At the same time, I had begun increasing my minimalist running gradually and started a new job where I wore high heels all day for a couple of days. I should have realized that switching between barefoot shoes and high heels was a really big difference and been more careful with that. It's tough because I wanted to look professional for my new job, and women's dress slacks are designed to be worn with heels only—they are too long to wear with flats. I didn't have time to try to come up with an alternative or get my pants tailored.

ciently recovered to do the next drill with good form. Your heart rate can get quite high in the short term while you're doing the drill and postdrill stride; allow it to lower before starting the next drill. After you've done the drill and postdrill strideout the second time, recover, then move on to the next exercise.

The order of the drills moves from gentlest to most challenging in terms of dynamic range of motion.

"I developed a weird top-of-foot injury. I'm not sure which variable caused it."

Another variable was that Cohen was returning to running after injury at this time. As she notes, "It's tricky because when you're beginning to run again after taking a break to heal, there are inevitable aches and pains that you have to run through as your body gets used to it again. It's tough to know what is a normal pain and what is the beginning of an injury."

Cohen's foot took months to feel better. During that time she developed a few guidelines for herself that most modern runners would do well to heed.

"The lesson definitely seems to be that for some people, going supergradual with all transitions is needed, and don't underestimate the importance of the casual time you spend on your feet when you're not running," she says. "I still want to get back to running in minimalist-ish shoes, although I am not committed to going all the way and only running in Merrells.

"I had thought that pure barefoot-style, zero-drop shoes were the only way to go and everything else was dumb and bad for you. But now I am realizing that, for some people, transitioning can take a really, really long time, and you might not be ready for that little of a shoe for a while, or ever, and that the in-between types of shoes can be really helpful. I also see the value in switching among several different types of shoes to make your feet stronger in a wider variety of situations and work them at different angles.

"I'm more committed now to being an all-around athlete and doing as many different activities as I can, because I hope it will help me be stronger, more flexible, and more resistant to injury, and it's fun to do new things!"

BACKWARD WALK

Backward walking activates the glutes and hamstrings.

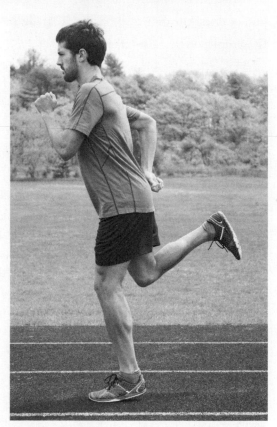

Why: This exercise activates the hamstrings and glute muscles so that you become more accustomed to using them to power the swing phase of your stride; the result is a stronger, more flowing stride than when you rely on the flexor muscles, such as the quadriceps, along the front of your body.

How: While staying on your forefoot, bend the leg you're going to lead with at the knee. Use your hamstrings and deep buttock muscles to extend that leg behind you. Walk backward as you continue to contract your glutes. Take long walking strides while keeping your upper body upright but relaxed. Cover 30 yards.

FAST-FEET SHUFFLE

Fast-feet shuffles improve stride frequency.

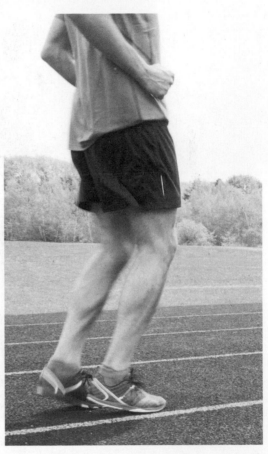

Why: This exercise will help improve your stride frequency by getting your nervous system used to firing more quickly. The shuffle can also help reduce a tendency to overstride. Finally, it works the peroneal muscles, on the outside of your lower legs; better activation of those muscles will help you get off your toes more quickly and with more power.

How: Staying on the balls of your feet, shuffle forward as quickly as you can while skimming over the ground just inches at a time. Keep your knee lift at a minimum. Keep your arms bent at a 90-degree angle and loose, and your torso upright and relaxed. Cover 10 yards. Proper recovery between drills is especially important with this exercise, so that your nervous system can fire as quickly as possible.

G DRILL

G drills lessen ground contact time.

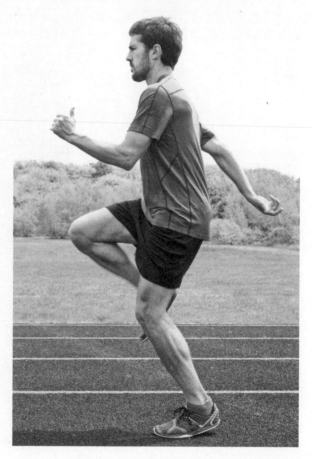

Why: This exercise will teach you how to get off the ground more quickly, thereby improving your stride rate and lessening the amount of time you spend in the stance phase of the running gait. It's especially helpful for runners whose feet splay out as they toe off.

How: Stand with one foot flat and the other leg bent at a 90-degree angle, with your arms in the appropriate corresponding positions. As quickly as possible, do an "exchange," getting into the same position on the other foot. While learning to do the drill, focus on doing 10 exchanges with the best balance possible. As you become better at the drill, see how many you can do with good balance in 15 seconds.

Butt Kick

Butt kicks improve the swing phase.

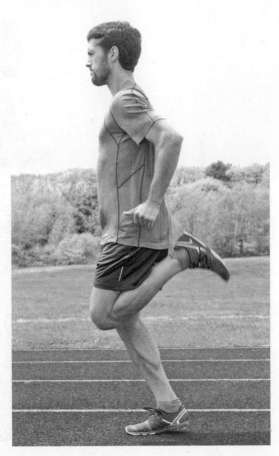

Why: This exercise helps to lessen the time it takes to bring your foot up and behind you after you toe off. It also teaches you to use your calf muscles more at toe-off and to keep your trail leg close to your backside rather than extended far behind you. Finally, it improves driving your arms quickly in sync with your legs.

How: While staying on your toes with your ankles dorsiflexed (feet pointed toward your shins), quickly snap your feet back to kick your butt. The first few times you do this drill, you might not be able to reach your butt; you should be able to with practice. Keep your head up and over your shoulders, and keep your upper body erect but not overly stiff. Although you want the foot-to-butt motion to be quick, don't worry about how swiftly you're moving across the ground. Cover 30 yards.

HIGH KNEE

High knees improve knee lift.

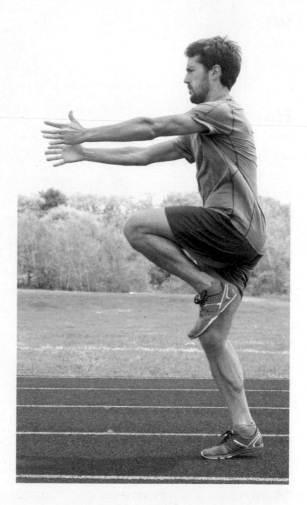

Why: This exercise works your quadriceps and hip flexors so that your knee lift is greater and more efficient.

How: Use a pistonlike motion to rapidly lift your knees and drive your toes back toward the ground. Stay on your toes throughout the drill. Hold your arms straight out in front of you as if you're carrying a pizza box; imagine trying to keep the box flat. It's okay to lean back a little if that helps with your knee lift. Cover 30 yards.

CARIOCA

Cariocas improve hip range of motion.

Why: This exercise works full range of motion in your hips.

How: If you're new to this drill, do it walking your first few times. Walk sideways, bringing your right foot in front of your left foot, then your right foot behind your left foot, repeating this pattern for 20 yards. Turn around and continue to walk sideways in the same direction, but now leading with your left leg—left foot in front of right foot, then left foot behind right foot, again repeating the pattern for 20 yards.

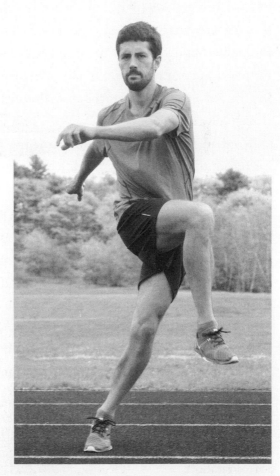

As the movement becomes familiar, convert the walk into a skip. Move laterally while swiveling your hips and swinging your arms across your body, alternately moving one leg behind your body, then bringing it across the front and lifting your knee high in the front swivel. Do 20 yards focusing on one leg, then turn 180 degrees and focus on the opposite leg for another 20 yards.

Over time the movement will feel more natural and you can concentrate on increasing the speed of the lateral skip and the distance you travel with each stride.

MODERN LIFE AND MINIMALISM

With age, many of us become increasingly removed from regularly moving through all planes of motion, as children tend to do while playing and participating in a wide variety of games and sports. At the same time, we tend to spend more and more time sitting, either in a car or at a desk. In the latter case, we're often slumped in front of a computer, perhaps with our head bent down and/or thrust forward.

None of this is good for our running form. Former Olympic marathoner and current office worker Pete Pfitzinger says that sitting all day at a desk means "the hamstrings become short and weak and the core muscles do not have to work as you lean back in your chair." Magill says, "It plays murder on our hips, and can also cause iliotibial band syndrome. Anything we do for a long time strains certain muscles, and they're going to go into spasm." Veteran coach Roy Benson adds, "As we spend less time being active and more time being passive, like sitting at a computer, even though we run, the less control we have of our skeleton by our muscular system, and that is a big problem." Wharton describes the effect of the sitting most of us do as "glutes in hibernation"— what should be the powerful muscles in your butt and hamstrings are rarely activated. Over time you lose the ability to use them effectively when running.

There are two modes of attack here—address the problems and prevent the problems. Addressing them includes regularly doing the strengthening exercises and drills outlined above. In addition, if you run after work, undo some of the day's damage with a dynamic warmup (leg swings, plus the milder drills, like backward walking) that will activate your running muscles and help you start the run with better form.

In addition to regular strengthening work, much of prevention comes down to day-to-day habits. Set up your monitor or other workstation so that it's at eye level. Move your monitor close enough so that you're not straining to see it (and therefore thrusting your head forward). Position your keyboard so that your elbows are bent at 90 degrees to minimize strain on your shoulders. When your shoulders and neck are tight and out of alignment, they'll throw off your hips, and your running form will suffer.

Sit with your center of gravity over your hips and your feet flat on the floor. Angle your chair so that your knees are slightly lower than your hips. (As much as possible, try to achieve the same posture while driving.) And no matter how good your sitting posture is, get up and move around at least once an hour to undo some of the chronic low-level strain on your shoulders, neck, and head.

Then there's the matter of what's on your feet during the vast majority of your life when you're not running.

Kevin Kirby, a sport podiatrist and marathoner in northern California, believes minimalists would do well to think about more than just their running shoes. "They are so worried about everyone's extra 8 millimeters of heel height during their 30- to 60-minute runs, but are saying nothing about the health effects that wearing shoes with 75 millimeters of heel height and overly tight toe boxes for 8 hours per day has on a woman's feet, knees, and lower back."

A British study published in 2010 documented the structural

changes that high heels cause. It measured gastrocnemius length and Achilles tendon agility in women who regularly wear high heels versus women who don't. The heel wearers' calf muscles were about 12 percent shorter, and their Achilles tendons were more than 10 percent more rigid than those of the women who wore flat shoes. As a result, the heel wearers had significantly less range of motion in their ankles.

A Finnish study published in 2012 showed how these sorts of structural changes have functional implications. Researchers gathered two groups: one made up of women who had worn heels of at least 5 centimeters for 40 hours a week for at least 2 years, and the other made up of women who wore heels for less than 10 hours a week. While the women walked over level ground, the researchers measured ankle and knee motion and lower-leg muscle activity. The heel wearers had measurable increases in fascial strain and muscle activity compared with the other group. Their history of wearing heels for much of the workweek had altered their basic walking mechanics. While the study looked at the effect of heels on walking, not running, it's reasonable to think the mechanical deficiencies would be that much more amplified when running.

Wearing flat shoes and going barefoot in sedentary hours is a key part of the transition-to-minimalism plan we looked at in Chapter 6. Continuing that practice is a key part of maintaining your running body. If heels are unavoidable in your profession, do the best you can to minimize the time you spend in them, such as wearing other shoes while commuting and taking the heels off when you know you'll be at your desk for a while.

MINIMALISM FOR YOUNG AND OLD

Parents used to be told their children should wear "supportive" shoes to help young feet adapt properly to increased activity. Fortunately, that thinking has been set aside by knowledgeable people. In running terms, most experts agree that young runners are ideal candidates for minimalist shoes, both because of less initial injury risk and because of the long-term gains to be had.

"I would encourage it for any adolescent," says Fullem. "My 10-year-old son just ran his first 5-K, and I try to get him in as minimalist a shoe as possible. I think if you start with the younger kids, their muscles and their tendons and everything get stronger."

"I think the high school kid should maybe push the envelope a little bit more in terms of minimalism," says Johnson, who conducts annual high school running camps in Boulder, Colorado. "I think sometimes kids get sold shoes that are made for heavier, middle-aged people training for a marathon when they're a light, waify kid whose longest race is 5-K." The "protection" that "supportive" shoes traditionally were said to provide should come via the strengthening work laid out earlier in this chapter, says Johnson.

Young runners have less injury risk running in minimal shoes because they haven't done years of mileage in bigger shoes that alter their mechanics and weaken and tighten key running muscles. For the same reason, they're also ideal candidates for extensive form work, says Steve Magness, a former coach with the Nike Oregon Project who's also worked with leading high school runners.

"They don't have years of 'This is how my running form is,'"

Magness says. "It's not ingrained as motor programming like with someone who's been running a long time. They're much more of a blank slate and easy to change with low risk." As Magness points out, young runners usually aren't doing much mileage, making their situation analogous to the start-from-scratch transition plan we looked at in Chapter 6.

"I'd generally go with a lightweight trainer for most high school kids," says Magness. "Not something crazy minimal, but more like what older runners might wear for long tempo runs and marathon-pace runs."

Johnson thinks that young runners will benefit from minimalism not only now, but also when they're adult runners. "We're at a really cool time in our country where kids are into the sport and the shoe companies are putting out 'less' shoes," he says. "I think we can have kids have fewer injuries in the next 10, 20 years as long as they're doing the strengthening work as well."

At the other end of the age-group spectrum, don't be dissuaded from running in minimalist shoes simply because you're middle-aged or older.

"All other things being equal, if you're an older runner, you should have better bone density than a sedentary person of your age," says Fullem. "It's known as Wolff's Law—your body responds to the stress of the pounding by strengthening the bone." You shouldn't be at a higher risk of stress fractures than younger runners from running in shoes with less cushioning.

If you're a new runner in your 40s or older and have been sedentary most of your life, then it's a good idea to have your bone density checked regardless of what shoes you run in.

As we saw in Chapter 6, younger new runners can sometimes

transition to minimalist shoes quicker than their contemporaries who have run for many years. If you're an older new runner and your bone density is good, you should be able to use minimalist shoes as one of your footwear options without undue concern for getting a stress fracture.

MINIMALISM IN YOUR ARSENAL

You're probably familiar with the fact that it's easier to maintain fitness than to obtain it. That principle also applies to improvements in your running form—once it's gotten better because of minimalist shoes, strengthening exercises, and drills, it's easier to run with good form in whatever shoes you wear. Certainly that's the experience of elite Kenyans, who grow up covering lots of miles in little or no shoes, and then maintain beautiful form once they start running in conventional shoes.

Of course, you need to be diligent about the strengthening work and form drills, especially if you have a typical Western lifestyle. But running in minimalist shoes isn't an all-or-nothing matter any more than most other aspects of running are. If you enjoy doing all your running in minimalist shoes, great. If you enjoy running in minimalist shoes and more conventional models, feel free to do so. You won't be kicked out of any club (at least any worth being part of). And you'll be putting into practice what successful runners have long done—rotating shoes.

Joe Rubio, coach of the Asics Aggies and a 2:18 marathoner at his prime, says, "I've been coaching a long time, and 80 to 85 percent of the people are going to have the most success alternating different shoes for different purposes. When I was really racing, you had spikes for really fast stuff, a really light pair of racing flats for 5-K race-pace workouts, a little more substantial shoe for tempo runs, a lightweight trainer for most of your regular runs, and a padded pair of bricks for your true recovery days, because you wanted to run slow and not take the pounding. And you did your barefoot strides.

"It's like interval training back in the '60s—you did it every frickin' day!" Rubio continues. "It worked for some people, but it didn't work for a huge number of people. In my mind, it's the same thing with real minimalist shoes. Some people can train in them for everything and be fine, but most people are going to do better by picking certain days to train in that type of footwear. They'll still get the advantages."

Many runners find that once they've become accustomed to running in less shoe, they no longer enjoy running in traditional trainers. (I'm one of them.) If that's you, consider rotating shoes within the minimalist spectrum. Popular minimalist blogger Peter Larson says, "If I had to pick three or four shoes, I'd probably want something with maybe a 4-millimeter heel rise and some decent cushioning for longer runs; a racing flat; something that has no cushioning as a training tool and for form work and shorter runs; and a trail shoe."

Larson, who teaches college courses in anatomy, points out a key value of shoe rotation beyond the performance aspects Rubio outlined above.

"If you ask me why injuries happen, I think it's because we run lots of miles on terrain that doesn't vary at all," Larson says. "And that's not necessarily because it's hard, but we go out and run on the road and there's no variation and we pound our legs in the same shoes on the same runs every single day and there's no variability. I haven't seen any studies comparing injury rates in trail runners versus road runners, but running on trails varies things. If you want to try to get that variation on the roads, running in a few different pairs of shoes might be one way to do that."

If you find you're a happy, healthy runner doing all your mileage in minimalist shoes, great. If you find you're a happy, healthy runner doing two runs a week in minimalists, or somewhere between that and all your running, that's great, too. There are no rules you have to follow about how often to wear minimalist shoes. Five years from now, you're more likely to be a healthy runner enjoying your sport if you avoid extremes and rigid but arbitrary standards. That applies to mileage, diet, competitive goals, stretching and strengthening, and pretty much everything else, including what shoes you choose to run in.

Five years from now, if you've made minimalism part of a sustainable approach to your running, what will your minimalist shoe choices be? That's the subject of our final chapter.

CHAPTER 9

MINIMALISM
IN THE LONG RUN

Where are minimalist
shoes headed?

AS THE PHYSICIST NIELS BOHR once said, perhaps while channeling Yogi Berra, prediction is very difficult, especially about the future. Who in 2005 would have predicted that 5 years later the Vibram FiveFingers would be the top seller in outdoor specialty retail sales? Or that shoes with massive heel heights like the Nike

Shox, which runners were then buying by the boatload, would soon be viewed as evil incarnate?

Still, it's fun and often educational to forecast how today's reality might morph into tomorrow's trends. In this chapter we'll get expert opinion on where minimalist shoes are heading. Will barely there shoes like the Vibram FiveFingers still be popular? Will minimalist shoes constitute more or less of the overall running-shoe market? Where are running shoes in general headed, and how might manufacturing innovations affect them and their relationship with minimalism? And finally, will the minimalist movement cause shoe manufacturers to throw out their traditional paradigm for designing shoes?

THINNING THE MINIMALIST HERD

As we saw in Chapter 5, minimalism encompasses a broad range of shoes, from barely there models like the FiveFingers and Merrell Trail Glove to moderate minimalists like the New Balance Minimus Road and Nike Free to gateway or transitional shoes like the Saucony Kinvara and Brooks PureConnect.

At the beginning of the decade, the barely there shoes were the hottest. Vibram had nudged its way into constituting 2 percent of running-shoe sales; that's a remarkable achievement for a brand that basically had 0 percent 5 years earlier. Solely because of Vibram, the big seven running-shoe companies—Nike, Asics, Adidas, New

Balance, Brooks, Saucony, and Mizuno—saw their traditional 96 percent share of the market slip to 94 percent. Vibram's market share might have gone even a little higher if the firm had been able to keep up with demand. In late 2009 and early 2010, the company was frantically adding staff and production facilities, but some stores still couldn't keep FiveFingers in stock. Sales were roughly doubling every year.

That growth trend has stopped. In the first quarter of 2012, according to industry analyst SportsOneSource.com, Vibram sales declined by more than half. That happened for two key reasons.

First, there are more choices now within the barefoot-style neighborhood of minimalism. Merrell has created a well-liked line of barely there road and trail shoes, niche brands like Vivobarefoot are more widely available, and the big players now have this ground covered if they so choose (for example, the Adidas Adipure Trainer, which features Vibramesque toe pockets).

Second, the pendulum that swung so quickly from traditional running shoes to the other extreme is now moving back. "I don't know how many people are buying a second or third pair of Five Fingers," says Joe Rubio, a partner in the online running store RunningWarehouse.com and one of the most astute industry watchers around.

"I think we may have reached the end of people's infatuation with them," says Peter Larson, author of the popular minimalist shoe blog Runblogger, about the FiveFingers. "The fit is so hard to get right. The toe pockets, you either love those or hate those when you run in them. I think a lot of them are sitting in people's closets." Regardless of its resolution, a spring 2012 proposed class-action lawsuit against Vibram for false advertising claims certainly symbolized a potential end of the love affair with the less-is-always-better approach.

"What we're going to see is a growth in the quasi-minimalist area," Larson says. "I think the no-cushion-at-all Merrell Trail Glove area will be a small part of the market. The majority of people are going to want some amount of cushion under their feet. I think the growth will be from the Kinvara type down to flat cushioned shoes like what Altra is producing."

Rubio says market realities will hasten the pendulum's swing away from the extreme end of minimalism.

"There was an argument after Vibrams got big that the big brands didn't want to do these minimal shoes," he says with a scoff. "Okay, if you're Brooks and you're looking at this whole thing and you've got an Adrenaline that has a three-piece medial post with all the plastic pieces in there . . . you know how expensive it is to make that shoe? Why would you want to make that shoe versus a one-piece midsole/outsole with no added technology? Your cost has got to be 60 percent of a traditional shoe, maybe less."

The result of big brands moving in, Rubio says, will be the death of some smaller ones. "Any big idea that the small brands come up with will migrate to the big brands, who have lots of resources and access to the end consumer," he says. "That makes it very hard for any of the small brands to gain significant traction in the market-place. You've got a bazillion small companies knocking it out for that final 4, 5 percent of the marketplace. Some of them are going to have to go away."

It's not so much that all the big companies will make shoes to compete toe-to-toe with the niche minimalist brands, but that their minimalist offerings will seem minimal enough to most runners.

That is, people who want only the FiveFingers will go looking for the FiveFingers, but people looking for "less shoe" will be much more likely to find the big brands' minimalist offerings and deny the smaller brands a chance at a sale. That's especially true if you consider Larson's point about growth in minimalism coming in the slightly cushioned segment instead of the barely there models, which tend to be made by the smaller companies. And then there's this: About 70 percent of sales within the minimalist category go to one shoe, the Nike Free.

In any industry, Rubio points out, economies of scale usually favor larger companies. In the running-shoe industry, he says, "The basics of the business are that a small company doesn't deliver necessarily on time, whereas a big company generally does. And if you're running a business, you need to have stuff show up on time. And what if something goes wrong with the product? A smaller company can't deal with a big blunder if they come up with a product that doesn't hit, whereas a big company can absorb it." Translation: If the Adidas Adipure Trainer doesn't take off, Adidas will survive. Niche brand Somnio invested heavily in a minimalist shoe, the Nada, that never made it to stores; the project helped drive the company from the US running market.

Rubio adds, "The big companies, just the sheer number of shoes they have to choose from is incredible. They have their traditional shoes, their minimal shoes, their racing flats, their trail shoes. Some of these little brands make only one or two models, and what if you don't like them?"

So a few of the many small companies that were making barefoot-style running shoes while I was writing this book might not exist by the time you're reading it. Will other companies follow the Skechers plan—use their deep pockets to develop a minimalist running shoe and try to make inroads into an industry they've not historically been part of? Skechers' first running shoe, the lightweight GoRun, has gotten mostly positive reviews from initially incredulous minimalists. The brand scored a coup by signing as their one sponsored runner Meb Keflezighi, who won the 2012 US Olympic Marathon Trial in Skechers.

Rubio is dubious. "Every 6 months you have another company that tries," he says. "We're not carrying Skechers [at Running Warehouse.com]. The guy keeps calling us asking why not. I say, 'I know you have Meb, and Meb's a friend of mine, but you got a crappy brand name. You got Kim Kardashian as a spokesperson. There's no credibility with that brand. You have a decent shoe, but until the brand name gets better, there's no point in carrying it.'

"If someone like Puma, with a tradition and decent product, can't sell shoes, no way can I see Skechers making it," Rubio continues. "If you're a brick-and-mortar store, why would you give up shelf space for something that might move versus something that is moving? And besides, how much room do I have in my back room to store this thing?"

The break-in brands then have to look for sales in what the industry calls "other channels," in this case meaning outside of specialty running stores and large sporting goods chains, or largely through online sales. Rubio says, "There aren't enough people looking for it in those other channels. The only thing in recent memory that made it that way is the FiveFingers. Long-term, you gotta get in brick-and-mortar."

MINIMALISM IN THE MARKET

If you paid attention only to news stories, you'd be excused for thinking that minimalist shoes are pretty much the only running shoes people have bought the last few years. And yes, in the spring of 2012, minimalist shoes were still hot, with sales increasing by 70 percent or more most months. But here's a reality check: In the first quarter of 2012, minimalist shoes accounted for about 11 percent of the US running-shoe market. Remove the Nike Free from consideration, and sales of the remaining minimalist models constituted 4 percent of the US market.

"It's similar to hybrid and electric cars," Rubio says. "There's a huge amount of press, and every ad you see touts these technologies, but if you look at the sales figures, it's 2 to 3 percent of the industry."

Rubio's livelihood depends on intimate knowledge of the US running-shoe scene. Ignoring hard data and what most people want simply isn't an option in his line of work. So I asked him what he thought would be the biggest sellers on RunningWarehouse. com in 2015.

"It'll still be traditional trainers," he says. "They make up 80 percent of our sales. In the industry as a whole, they're more like 90 percent of sales.

"There are two customers in the processes: the people who sell the shoes and the public. The people selling running shoes to the customer, they need to make business decisions more on what's definitely going to work versus what might work. And the guys who are making the shoes for the dealers are only going to respond by making what's popular. So I don't see minimalism getting any bigger than it is now."

But what about all the press for minimalism? I asked. Aren't customers influenced by that, and wouldn't that change what they ask for when shopping for running shoes?

"The people going to brick-and-mortar tend to be the people at the last third of the race, the beginning athlete who needs a lot of guidance," Rubio responds. "They might have heard about this FiveFingers thing, and they might buy a pair. And maybe they'll do as recommended and start off walking around or hiking in them, and go, 'Wow, this is a lot of work and kind of painful, versus my [Asics] Nimbus, which are really comfortable and plush and they look good and I can go out afterward in them.' There's always going to be a place for traditional shoes that are soft and comfortable and look good."

When considering minimalism's share of the overall market, it's helpful to keep in mind where most running shoes are sold. Sixty percent of sales occur in department stores like Nordstrom. Thirty percent are through what the industry calls "big box"— large chains like Sports Authority or Dick's Sporting Goods. Only 10 percent are through running specialty stores or online outfits like Rubio's.

"The final 10 percent is where a lot of the smaller brands would hope to get shelf space," Rubio says. "No way Nordstrom brings in a small, unknown but trending brand."

Most running-shoe sales occur elsewhere than what most readers of this book would consider a good place to buy running shoes. Because of this simple market reality, it's hard for knowledgeable industry watchers like Rubio to see minimalist shoes making inroads beyond their current share of about 10 percent of sales. And yet . . .

BEYOND CATEGORY

"They're hugely influential," Rubio says of the minimalist shoes it might seem he's just been deriding. "If you look at things that are happening in the auto industry, you're seeing Porsches that get 72 miles per gallon for the fastest production car they've ever made. The same thing's happening in the running industry. You've got these really lightweight minimal shoes that are having a huge influence on how all shoes are made."

That influence is showing in two key aspects of running-shoe construction: weight and ramp angle, or the difference between heel and forefoot height. For example, after the tremendous success of the Kinvara, with its reported 4-millimeter ramp angle, Saucony is lowering the heel-to-toe differential throughout its line from 12 millimeters to 8 millimeters. Combine that with less weight, and you might find yourself asking, Is this a conventional shoe? A minimalist model? What?

"I think the movement toward lighter and faster and more responsive isn't going to end," says Rubio. "It's just going to be a natural part of shoe development. It's similar to the bike industry, where you gotta keep making things lighter every year. Any one bike from year to year might not be significantly different, but over the course of 5 years, you notice a pretty big change in the weight and responsiveness. Every industry goes lighter over time. I'm just surprised it took running this long to get there."

The gains in lightness are coming not only from minimalist-driven consumer demand. They're also driven by improvements in manufacturing processes that would be lowering shoe weight regardless of whether models like the FiveFingers had ever become popular.

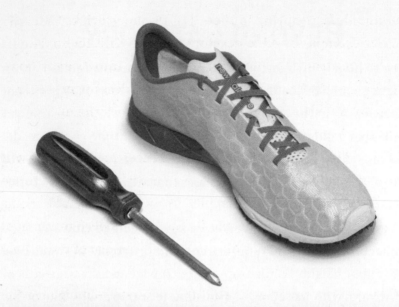

At just over 3 ounces, the New Balance RC 5000 weighs the same as this small screwdriver.

"There are so many new materials being created over in Asia that are superlightweight, superstrong, superresilient," says Brian Metzler, a former *Running Times* senior editor who's wear-tested more than 1,000 shoes. "So whatever you need a piece of a shoe to do, whether it's add stretchiness for comfort or add firmness, there are these new materials playing a huge role in the shoe revolution."

New manufacturing processes, like welding instead of stitching, will lead to lighter shoes, Metzler says. Welding ultrathin synethic overlays instead of sewing heavier ones is one reason why New Balance was able to make a racing flat, the RC 5000, weigh in at just 3.3 ounces when it was released in the summer of 2012. Lighter shoes will also happen as companies move from "heavier overlays and various plastics and vinyls that weren't really that conducive to a running shoe, resulting in these 14-, 15-ounce bricks," Metzler says. For example, as Nike developed its Fly Knit technology, it found lessons from that process it could carry into its entire running-shoe line. By trying to create a snug, seamless upper—a development unrelated to minimalism—Nike found a way for all its shoes to lose 10 percent of their weight.

As such developments happen, differences among shoes will become more a matter of degree than category. "You'll start to see some of these categories overlapping," says Metzler. "Take racing flats—now you see a lot of people wearing the modern minimalist shoes, like the New Balance Minimus Road, instead of traditional racing flats."

Rubio sees the lines blurring most in the already-ambiguous distinction between basic training shoe and lightweight trainer. "Now you get a [Nike] Pegasus under 10 ounces, so an everyday training shoe starts moving toward what we would have called a lightweight trainer a few years ago," he says. "Something like the New Balance 890, an everyday trainer, not a minimalist shoe, that's significantly lighter—that's where I think you'll see things going. Brands that aren't doing that are losing sales significantly."

MOVING PAST THE PRONATION PARADIGM

For the last couple of decades, the model for conceiving and designing running shoes has been based largely on pronation control. The thinking has been that what happens to your foot as it hits the ground is what's most important. If your foot rolls in a little between landing and pushing off, you're said to have normal pronation, and have been told to go with a "neutral" shoe, sort of the Goldilocks version of running shoes—not too soft, not too rigid, providing just the right amount of cushioning and stability. If your foot rolls in too much, we've

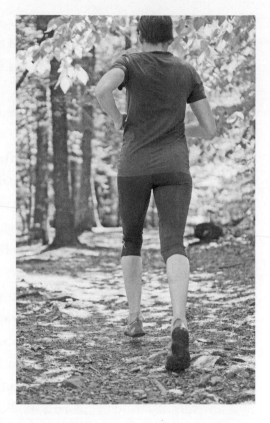

been told, you need a motion-control shoe that will arrest some of the overpronation. And if your foot barely rolls in but instead remains rigid upon landing, you're said to be an underpronator, or supinator, and therefore need a flexible, cushioned shoe to absorb some of the shock that would be dissipated if you had a normal amount of pronation.

The minimalist movement has led an increasing number of people throughout running to question this model. Many runners who were told to wear stiff, heavy motion-control shoes have felt liberated (and remained injury-free) by moving to barely there shoes that allow their feet to work naturally. Sales in the motion-control category of running shoes have been in decline the last few years, and good riddance to all that, say many running experts.

"One of the things with the traditional line that you'll probably see—and are already starting to see—is the dissolution of the pronation-control category," says minimalist blogger and college biology professor Peter Larson. "There's never really been evidence supporting those, and in fact there's now research that came out recently showing that those don't work."

Here Larson is referring to studies such as one with Marines that followed the traditional practice of assigning shoe type based on arch height; the study found little effect on incidence of injury even after other injury factors were considered. Even more interesting, a Canadian study randomly assigned three types of shoes—neutral, stability or motion-control—to a group of women runners. The researchers found that there was no relationship between the type of shoe the women wore and their incidence of running-induced pain. That is, women who were "supposed" to be in motion-control shoes reported as much or more pain when wearing those shoes as did women who were "supposed" to be in motion-control shoes but were in one of the other, supposedly less suitable types. "The findings of this study suggest that our current approach of prescribing in-shoe pronation control systems on the basis of foot type is overly simplistic and potentially injurious," the researchers concluded.

Steve Magness, formerly an assistant coach with the Nike Oregon Project and holder of a master's degree in exercise sciences, agrees, noting, "I think in the lab you're seeing more of the thought that this model probably doesn't work, so let's come up with another theory." Magness likes to point out that the focus on pronation came about at least as much because it could be measured in the lab as because those measurements yielded meaningful data.

"The question is, Do you keep using a model that most people think is broken just because it's what we've always done?" asks Larson. "What do we do instead? There you kinda get stuck. That's a huge question right now, and I wish I had the answer."

Indeed, it's difficult to see how the great running insight "we're all an experiment of one" can be matched with modern industry's penchant for flow charts and categorization. Which company is more likely to get the average consumer's purchase: one whose promotional materials provide quick, easy guidance on navigating their product line, or one that more or less admits "your guess is as good as ours"? As Magness says, "We know different shoes work for different people based on a couple of different things. But how do we translate that into designing shoes and classifying shoes?"

Consider flat feet, says Larson. Under the pronation-control model, nearly everyone with flat feet has been put in motion-control shoes, because the assumption has been that flat feet are prone to overpronation. As it turns out, "there are different reasons why people can have flat feet," Larson says, "so just putting everyone with a flat foot in one type of shoe doesn't make any sense. We're learning that flat feet when you're standing might not mean anything about what the foot does when you're running."

Magness, a voracious consumer of research, offers another

example: "With muscle activity, what they find is some people, if they have a lot of activity in their calves and their calves are really tight before footstrike, it makes them more economical," he says. "Some people it's the exact opposite. The question is why and what makes people different, and does that mean they need a different shoe? Would someone who relies entirely on reactive elastic response in their calves and Achilles need a really hard shoe that lets that work, where someone who doesn't rely on it, maybe they need a soft shoe to take some of the load?"

The muscle-activity thinking stems from the work of the Canadian biomechanist Benno Nigg, a professor at the University of Calgary. If the conventional paradigm considers running shoes the primary actor, a piece of equipment that gets the body to do what it's "supposed" to do, Nigg represents the opposite end: He believes footwear shouldn't affect footstrike, or even muscle activity before the foot hits the ground.

Good luck systematizing that in a way that can lead to mass production in Asian factories and helpful guidance in American stores, all at prices runners are accustomed to. And, notes Magness, even if this X factor could be isolated, it will be hard to keep its value in perspective. "We can measure pronation easily, so that's what everything is based on," he says. "There's going to be this shift of, well, maybe we can measure this other new thing really well, so let's make everything entirely based on that.

"The reality is, what people need in a running shoe is probably from some crazy combination of foot mechanics and pronation and muscle activity and structure," Magness says. "It's hard to tease out all these things and say, 'All right, here's the perfect combination.'"

THE ROAD AHEAD

"I fear that I may have been too negative in this attack, but there are times when a pendulum has swung far enough and needs a strong push in the other direction to restore equilibrium."

That's the famous evolutionary biologist Richard Dawkins in his book *Unweaving the Rainbow*. Although he was writing about how science gets taught, Dawkins's desire for restoring balance happens in most matters where people have passionate beliefs. A movement bursts on the scene, spearheaded by the most ardent and committed members. People are impressed by the purity of the message and the clear direction it provides on how to act. The newest recruits become some of the strongest proponents. Seemingly overnight, what had been obscure becomes common knowledge, and what the new movement is reacting against is seen as the folly of a less enlightened time.

Over time, however, most people find that the new movement pushed the pendulum too far. Through experimentation and going about their lives, people find what's most useful from the movement's message. What's helpful, they keep; what's not, they begin to ignore. The pendulum starts to move back to the center.

Have the movement's efforts been a waste? Most people would say no—through the process of the pendulum swing, they changed what's considered normal. Vegans get people to reconsider their use of animal products. Environmentalists make recycling mainstream. Back-to-the-landers show suburban homeowners the pleasure of a small garden plot. And, yes, hardcore minimalists get regular runners to reconsider what they run in.

The more extreme end of the minimalist movement was a necessary corrective. Although some runners were, on their own, finding a way around the ever-bigger shoes of the 1990s and early 2000s, most accepted the conventional line that if some cushioning is good, more is better. It took that big push of the pendulum to bring the issue of footwear fundamentals into the mainstream.

But Dawkins's quote applies to both ends of the pendulum's arc. As we've seen, that first pendulum swing is now over, and things are moving back to homeostasis. It's a new homeostasis, however, one that incorporates the minimalist message of running shoes serving the runner, rather than the other way around. That's been my belief throughout my 3-plus decades as a runner. I hope this book has helped you see the wisdom of that view and shown you how to implement it in your running in a way that works for you in the real world.

A MINIMALISM GLOSSARY

Here are some key words and phrases you'll encounter in this book.

BARELY THERE/BAREFOOT-STYLE SHOE

The most minimal of minimalist running shoes. These shoes generally have little to no cushioning between your foot and the outsole, and a slight stack height. As such, running in them replicates barefoot running better than running in other shoes, while providing protection from surface hazards. Most runners who have done the bulk of their lifetime mileage in conventional running shoes will need a slow, gradual transition to be able to run in barely there/barefoot-style shoes without risking injury.

BIOMECHANICS

How the parts of your body work together to create movement. In running, the term is sometimes used synonymously with running form, but it's more accurate to say that your biomechanics determine what your running form looks like. When you develop the needed strength and flexibility, running in minimalist shoes or barefoot can improve your biomechanics and thereby improve your running form.

DUAL-DENSITY MIDSOLE

A shoe-construction method in which the midsole is firmer in one section than elsewhere; usually, the firmer section is on the inside, near the heel.

The idea is that the harder part of the midsole helps to control overpronation better. Dual-density midsoles are anathema to most minimalists, who say such midsoles make conventional running shoes that much more likely to interfere with the foot's natural motion.

FOREFOOT STRIKE

Landing with the front of your foot first when running. A true forefoot strike at normal running speed (as opposed to racing) is rare, but switching to minimalist shoes and working on running form can move many runners away from heavy heel-striking and encourage them to use their forefoot more effectively.

GROUND CONTACT TIME

How long your foot stays on the ground when you're running. A longer ground contact time is generally associated with slower turnover, and it increases deceleration as you move through the gait cycle. Running barefoot or in minimalist shoes tends to lessen runners' ground contact time and can retrain your nervous system to run this way even when you're in more conventional running shoes.

HEEL COUNTER

The part of a running shoe that wraps around the back of your foot. Minimalist shoes tend to have a more flexible heel counter than conventional running shoes to encourage more natural foot motion. Some models' heel counters are collapsible.

HEEL STRIKE

Landing with your heel first when running. Although heel-striking isn't inherently bad, minimalists contend that modern running shoes can cause people who wouldn't heel-strike when running barefoot to do so when running shod. Most experts agree that too much of a heel strike can be a source of injury and poorer performance.

HEEL-TO-TOE DROP

The difference between a shoe's stack height in the heel and its stack height at the lowest point of the forefoot. Minimalists contend that shoes with too great a heel-to-toe drop encourage severe heel-striking and inhibit the calf muscles and Achilles tendons from working through their full range of motion.

MEDIAL POST

An addition of firmer material along the inside of a shoe's midsole, usually near the heel. Medial posts are supposed to help control overpronation. Minimalists contend that, rather than helping runners avoid injury, medial posts usually keep your feet and lower legs from working naturally and can increase your risk of injury.

MIDFOOT STRIKE

Move accurately called "flat-footed striking," or landing with the heel and forefoot at the same time. Midfoot-striking is less common than heel-striking but more common than forefoot-striking. Many runners find that, by switching to minimalist shoes and working on their running form, over time they adopt more of a midfoot strike. This, in turn, can mean less impact force and, many runners say, simply makes their stride feel more flowing.

MIDSOLE

The part of a running shoe between the outsole and upper. Conventional running shoes tend to have thick, cushioned midsoles. Minimalists contend that the midsoles in modern running shoes interfere with natural running mechanics because they're too soft, too high off the ground, and too tilted forward. Minimalist shoes tend to have firmer, lower, and flatter midsoles.

MINIMALISM

The belief that lighter, flatter, more flexible shoes allow people to run more like they're running barefoot than do conventional running shoes and thereby improve their running form and reduce their injury risk. For more details, read the preceding nine chapters!

MODERATE MINIMALIST SHOE

A shoe with construction features between a transitional minimalist shoe and a barefoot-style/barely there shoe. Moderate minimalist shoes have some midsole cushioning and a greater stack height than barely there models but are still a marked change for runners accustomed to conventional running shoes.

ORTHOTICS

Devices, often customized, put inside running shoes in the hope of preventing or overcoming injury. Most minimalists say that runners should wean themselves off orthotics and let the feet and lower legs learn how to run naturally. Sport podiatrists tend to agree that orthotics should be considered part of the fix for an acute situation rather than a lifelong presence, but they also think that runners can increase their injury risk if they abandon prescription orthotics too hastily.

OUTSOLE

The part of the shoe that contacts the running surface and provides traction and stability. Most minimalist shoes have a relatively level outsole to maximize the foot's ability to feel and adapt to the running surface. Minimalist trail shoes usually have a heavier, more lugged outsole than minimalist road shoes so that you don't feel every rock and twig on the trail.

OVERSTRIDING

Landing with the heel far out in front of the body. Note that overstriding has to do with foot position on landing, not stride length. Runners can have long stride lengths but not overstride. Most runners find it almost impossible to overstride while running barefoot. Wearing minimalist shoes, increasing functional strength and flexibility, and being mindful of running form can help overcome a tendency to overstride.

PRONATION

Rolling in of the foot after landing. Almost all runners pronate. One of the guiding ideas behind conventional running shoes is that too much pronation leads to injury and needs to be controlled by shoes; models built to control overpronation are heavier and stiffer than most other running shoes. Most experts now agree that overpronation as a driving factor in shoe design is a bad idea, and minimalists believe that motion-control shoes do much more harm than good.

RACING FLAT

A shoe designed to be worn in road races. Most racing flats have little heel-to-toe drop, a relatively small midsole, little cushioning, and an out-sole built more for traction than for durability. Competitive runners have long worn racing flats during their faster workouts, and many minimalists do much of their running in racing flats. One drawback to wearing racing flats for daily running is that some flats wear out more quickly than shoes designed specifically as minimalist shoes.

RAMP ANGLE

The angle formed by the difference between a shoe's stack height in the heel and its stack height at the lowest point of the forefoot. Minimalists contend that shoes with too great a ramp angle encourage severe heel-striking and inhibit the calf muscles and Achilles tendons from working through their full range of motion. A given model's ramp angle usually differs among various shoe sizes because most models have the same heel-to-toe drop regardless of how long the shoe is; hence, smaller shoe sizes usually have a steeper ramp angle than larger sizes.

STACK HEIGHT

A measurement of everything between the bottom of your foot and the top of the road, including the midsole and outsole. Heel-to-toe drop (or ramp angle) is calculated from the stack height. For example, a shoe with a stack height of 19 millimeters in the heel and 15 millimeters in the forefoot has a heel-to-toe drop of 4 millimeters. Generally speaking, minimalists contend that the greater a shoe's stack height, the greater the chance the midsole cushioning will interfere with how you run barefoot; the reasons given include that a large amount of cushioning does some of the work your feet and lower legs are designed to do, and too much material between your feet and your running surface introduces instability.

STRIDE RATE

The number of steps you take per minute while running. Stride rate—also called turnover—is usually expressed as the total number of steps both feet take in a minute. Stride rate varies to some degree with your pace (higher stride rate at faster paces). Although there's no ideal stride rate, most experts advise working toward a stride rate of 170 or more for moderate-paced and faster running; stride rates of 160 or less usually indicate overstriding. Most runners find that their stride rate increases at least a few steps a minute when they run barefoot or in minimalist shoes.

TOE BOX

The area at the front of a running shoe that houses your toes. Most conventional running shoes taper toward the front. This construction can cramp toes and prevent them from spreading as you land and push off, as occurs when you run barefoot. Many minimalist shoes have a wider-than-average toe box that allows more natural foot motion.

TOE SHOES

Running shoes with a separate "pocket" or container for each toe: Vibram FiveFingers are the most popular. Proponents of toe shoes contend that this construction best allows the toes to work as they do when you run barefoot. Some minimalist runners say a satisfying fit can be difficult if one's toes aren't the same length as the separate pockets.

TOE SPRING

The upward curvature of a running shoe at the front. Toe spring is usually more pronounced in conventional running shoes than in minimalist models. Many minimalists look for shoes with not much toe spring on the theory that too much toe spring inhibits the toes' ability to flatten and spread naturally and encourages more heel-striking. But because most minimalist shoes have a more flexible midsole than conventional running shoes, what might look like a large toe spring becomes functionally not as much of a factor as it would be in shoes with a stiffer construction.

TRANSITIONAL/GATEWAY SHOE

A shoe designed to ease a runner's transition into minimalism. These models maintain many features of conventional running shoes, including a relatively high midsole and relatively soft cushioning, while having a lower heel-to-toe drop than most running shoes. Although minimalist purists might scoff at transitional shoes, many runners find them helpful in learning how to better use their feet and lower legs while avoiding the soreness that can accompany a too-sudden switch to lighter, lower minimalist models. Many runners happily stop their minimalism journey at transitional shoes.

UPPER

The part of a running shoe that covers the top of the foot. Most minimalist shoes have a light, spare upper designed only to secure the foot to the rest of the shoe. The overlays and thick padded tongues found in the uppers of many conventional running shoes add weight and interfere with the foot's natural motion, minimalists contend.

ZERO-DROP SHOE

A shoe that has a heel-to-toe drop (or ramp angle) of 0; the heel and forefoot stack heights are the same. Proponents of zero-drop shoes say this construction allows the feet and lower legs to work like they do when running barefoot. Most runners need to work gradually toward running in zero-drop shoes to minimize their risk of calf and Achilles soreness or injury. A zero-drop shoe can still provide a lot of cushioning, depending on its stack height.

ONLINE MINIMALISM RESOURCES

The Web is awash with materials on minimalism. The short list below focuses on resources that value the tenets of minimalism while avoiding stridency and maintaining perspective on how the modern minimalist movement fits in with running history and the larger running world.

RUNNING TIMES' MINIMALIST CHANNEL

Running Times has been a leader in presenting real-world information on the merits of minimalism. The magazine's minimalist channel (running times.com/minimalism) contains several articles with use-at-home information on topics like how to know if you're ready for minimalism, how to make the transition safely, and how to make sure shoes fit properly to allow natural foot movement. There are also a lot of shoe reviews collected there.

COLLECTED MINIMALISM RESEARCH LINKS

As mentioned in Chapter 4, I've collected the most important research on minimalism-related topics such as foot strike, injury rates, and shoe type at runnersworld.com/minimalismlinks. There you'll find a brief description of the main findings of each study listed and a link to its abstract or full text, depending on the policy of the journal in which the study appeared.

PETER LARSON'S BLOG: RUNBLOGGER

Peter Larson, whose thoughts you'll find throughout this book, is a professor of biology at St. Anselm College in New Hampshire and is the coauthor of the book *Tread Lightly*. He maintains a deservedly popular blog that's mostly about minimalism at runblogger.com. Larson's blog frequently highlights new minimalism-related research; his posts do an excellent job of explaining a certain study and putting it in context given what other studies on similar matters have found. Larson is also an enthusiastic shoe collector who provides extensive wear-test reports on most minimalist shoes soon after—or sometimes before—they hit the market.

STEVE MAGNESS'S BLOG: THE SCIENCE OF RUNNING

Steve Magness, another source for this book, is the cross-country coach at the University of Houston and a former assistant coach under Alberto Salazar at the Nike Oregon Project. A 4:01 miler in high school, Magness has a master's degree in exercise science and is an inveterate consumer of physiology research. At his blog, scienceof running.com, he combines his coaching and athletic experience with his education to provide real-world takes on running, including, frequently, shoe choice and running form. Given his background and interests, Magness's analysis of research often centers on whether a given approach will answer what are most runners' two most important questions: Will this help me run faster and will this keep me from getting injured?

ROSS TUCKER'S AND JONATHAN DUGAS'S BLOG: THE SCIENCE OF SPORT

Ross Tucker and Jonathan Dugas each have a PhD in exercise science; they cowrite the blog sportscientists.com. Their interests are wide ranging, but they write frequently about running. Their posts on footwear and barefoot running are models of balancing experience and research and placing studies that others trumpet as game changers in proper context. Authors of the book *The Runner's Body,* Tucker, and Dugas are also adept at showing how topics like running form relate to the bigger picture of what happens to our bodies when we run ambitiously.

ALEX HUTCHINSON'S BLOG: SWEAT SCIENCE

Alex Hutchinson has represented Canada in international competition, and he has a PhD in physics. He knows how to read scientific literature, assess its positives and shortcomings, and describe its relevance to runners. At his blog, sweatscience.runnersworld.com, Hutchinson often writes about studies done on injury rates, running form, and footwear.

RUNNER'S WORLD FORUMS

On the *Runner's World* site, there are two popular forums where runners of all backgrounds and abilities discuss all things minimalism: the Barefoot Running forum (runnersworld.com/barefoot-forums) and the Shoes forum (runnersworld.com/shoes-forums).

ACKNOWLEDGMENTS

PHIL LATTER PROVIDED THOUGHTFUL reading of the chapters at draft stage and reporting for a section of Chapter 6.

Phil Wharton, Steve Magness, Brian Fullem, Joe Rubio, Peter Larson, Jay Johnson, and Pete Magill freely shared their knowledge and time.

Jeff Dengate provided a thorough and insightful read at the layout stage.

Dave Kayser trusted me with his babies, otherwise known as the old shoes seen in Chapter 3.

Amby Burfoot and Frank Brooks gave helpful advice during difficult writing patches.

Robert Gomez (a 2:23 marathoner) and Julia Kirtland (the 1997 national marathon champion) were patient and willing models.

Eric Alexander and Steve Davis make music that revives flagging spirits.

Stacey Cramp worked her usual photographic magic and, when not holding a camera, gave above-and-beyond spousal support.

ABOUT THE AUTHOR

SCOTT DOUGLAS IS NEWS EDITOR for *Runner's World* and a former editor of *Running Times*. He's the author or coauthor of five other running books, including *Advanced Marathoning*. Douglas has run more than 100,000 miles since taking up the sport as a teen in 1979. He lives in South Portland, Maine.

INDEX

Boldface page references indicate illustrations.
Underscored references indicate boxed text.